Praise for Jon Gabriel and

THE GABRIEL METHOD

...I cannot thank you enough for assisting me in "flicking my thin switch back on."...I've not dieted for 2 weeks and lost 15.5 pounds.... I'd like to thank you from the bottom of my heart.

—Sarah Toohey

I find the most powerful parts are the visualization and mental aspects you teach.... Your book has been a revelation as far as explaining why I have had trouble losing weight.... I have lost about 15 pounds so far, and I now have a plan that I know...will get me long-term results without as much pain.

—Dave Parkes

I have lost another 3 pounds this week, despite indulging my cravings for chocolate. Fifty-five pounds total so far! I'm feeling better and better every day, and I have no loose skin! Thanks so much.... You inspire me every day!

—Denise Bullen

I bought your book last Monday and it is AMAZING. People like you really do make an impact on the world. You have covered the very thing that everyone else misses—the mind–body connection.

—Jodi Bell

Finally, a book that deals with the root causes of why people hang on to the fat.

—Nicola Allen

I have been reading your book...and gradually implementing the recommendations you make.... So far I've lost around 20 to 22 pounds within about seven weeks.

—David Buchbinder

I lost 113 pounds in about six months and I've kept it off for a year now. Also, my blood sugar levels went from a dangerously high 19 down to 6. I'm now within the normal range. They say I still have diabetes but I don't think I do.

—Amanda Pierce

I have read your book and love the concept. I have been going down the natural, organic path for a while now and have already lost 44 pounds just by NOT dieting and [by] eating foods closer to the earth. . . . I . . . truly believe you have found the key. . . . I gave up smoking two and a half years ago following a very similar concept . . . mind power as opposed to will power. . . . The mind is very powerful—thanks for writing this book.

—Tanya Faulkner

I have often thought that there was so much more to weight loss than counting calories. I often thought that emotional issues played a big part in weight gain/loss, but finding help with these issues was difficult until I read your book. Thanks you so much for all of the work that you have done so people like me can finally get the help that we need. You are truly an inspiration.

—Jacinta O'Leary

I cannot believe how much I'm not hearing food calling to me!! I'm craving good food just like you told me I would, and . . . I now look at my body and know it's already working hard to become the body I want and need it to be.

—Alison dall Stosic

I am astounded at the difference [your method] has made to my life. I have lost 15 pounds so far, and I just don't have the hunger pains I always used to have. . . . It really does work. . . . It is just too easy. Thank you so much for sharing your story with the world. I will be spreading the word.

—Melinda Clarke

THE GABRIEL METHOD

The Revolutionary **DIET-FREE** Way to Totally Transform Your Body

THE GABRIEL METHOD

Jon Gabriel

ATRIA BOOKS
New York London Toronto Sydney

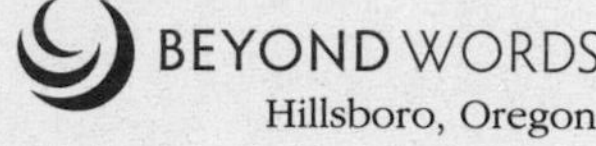

Hillsboro, Oregon

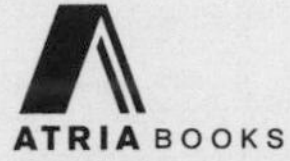
ATRIA BOOKS
A Division of Simon & Schuster, Inc.
1230 Avenue of the Americas
New York, NY 10020

BEYOND WORDS
20827 N.W. Cornell Road, Suite 500
Hillsboro, Oregon 97124-9808
503-531-8700 / 503-531-8773 fax
www.beyondword.com

The information contained in this book is intended to be educational and not for diagnosis, prescription, or treatment of any health disorder whatsoever. This information should not replace consultation with a competent healthcare professional. The content of this book is intended to be used as an adjunct to a rational and responsible healthcare program prescribed by a professional healthcare practitioner. The author and publisher are in no way liable for any misuse of the material.

Managing editor: Lindsay S. Brown
Editors: Gretchen Stelter, Xavier Waterkeyn
Proofreader: Jennifer Weaver-Neist
Design: Sara E. Blum
Composition: William H. Brunson Typography Services

First Atria Books/Beyond Words trade paperback edition January 2009

Manufactured in the United States of America

10 9 8 7 6 5

Library of Congress Cataloging-in-Publication Data:

Gabriel, Jon.
The Gabriel method : the revolutionary diet-free way to totally transform your body / Jon Gabriel.
p. cm.
1. Weight loss—Psychological aspects. I. Title.
RM222.2.G324 2008
613.2′5—dc22

2008030009

ISBN-13: 978-1-58270-218-6
ISBN-10: 1-58270-218-7

The corporate mission of Beyond Words Publishing, Inc.: *Inspire to Integrity*

To Inge

A child comes into this world bearing gifts.
The gifts you have given me have been beyond
my wildest imagination.

Contents

PART IV
Positive Forces that Make Your Body *Want* to Be Thin

PART V
Making It Happen for You

Acknowledgments

After having written and rewritten page after page, I now find the following paragraphs to be the hardest. Whenever I try to express my feelings about the love and support I've received from so many friends and family members, I am overcome with emotion.

So let me just say thank you—

To Sharon Humphreys; Xavier Waterkeyn; Rafael Nasser; Hilary Gans; Jack Strom; Uziel Silber; Eli Catalan; Ayesha Fletcher; Susan Correia; Chris and Angelika Hill; Khaliah Ali; Daphne Goldberg; An Soutar; Jeremy Longley; Jacqui Hellyer; Jude Tulloch; Anne Grieves; Alex Van Galen; Michelle Shilkin; Jasmine Jones; Clare Calvet; Robin Moran; Nancy Packs; Roydn Sweet; Louise Anderton; Nancy Nasser; James Nasser; Robert and Dongmei Peng; Phan; SP; Graham Hodges; Ashrita Furhman; Ananda Moy Ma; Lakshmi; and Jennifer, Michelle, Joseph, Ethel, and Leonard Abrams.

I have no other words to adequately express my appreciation.

I'd also like to thank the professional services of Tobin Dorn, Kelly Jones, Artha Holmes, Design Images, Denise Teo, Allen Cornwell, Courtney Dunham, Lindsay Brown, Marie Hix, Cynthia Black, Mellisa Radman, Greg Dinkin, Lyn Savage, and Grant Lewers.

And special thanks to Emma, Debra, Nari, Ruth, Helmi, Lisa, and Oona for creating flow in every area of my work and life.

Introduction: My Own Transformation

The Gabriel Method is the revolutionary new DIET-FREE way to get fit by getting your body to want to be thin.

I distinctly remember the moment that changed my life forever. It happened in August of 2001. I weighed close to 410 pounds. Over the previous twelve years, I had gained more than 200 pounds.

I had just gotten off Route 4 in New Jersey at the Paramus / River Edge exit. As I was getting off the exit, a thought stunned me like an electric shock: "My body wanted to be fat, and as long as it *wanted* to be fat, there was nothing I could do to lose weight." I turned onto the nearest side street and just sat there in my car.

Not another thought came into my head for the next twenty minutes.

During the twelve years in which I gained two hundred pounds, I had tried everything I could to lose weight, including every diet under the sun—from low-fat diets to low-carb diets and everything in between. I had spent time at both Nathan Pritikin's institute in California and with the late Dr. Atkins himself in New York.

I spent over three thousand dollars with Dr. Atkins, and in the end, the best he could do was yell at me for being so fat. I also spent several other small fortunes on every conceivable holistic cure and alternative health treatment available. No matter what I did, my body continued to gain weight.

Every diet or program I went on always followed the exact same pattern. It started with my having to count something—calories, fat, carbohydrates, salt, whatever—and a list of things I could not have. I followed the diet to the letter. I usually lost weight quickly in the beginning, but then the rate at which I lost weight would start to slow. Eventually, I stopped losing weight altogether. At that point, I was dieting, not to lose weight, but simply to maintain my current weight.

All the while my cravings for the foods that I was not allowed to have escalated. Discouraged and dejected, there would come a time when I was just too exhausted to fight my cravings anymore, and I would binge. Weight that had taken me a month or so to lose came back in just a matter of days. A few weeks later, I was invariably 10 to 15 pounds heavier than when I had started the diet.

No matter what I did to try to lose weight, my body fought me tooth and nail, and in the end, it always won. After years of banging my head against the wall and trying to force myself to lose weight, I had to concede that, as long as my body wanted to be fat, the situation was hopeless.

From the moment I made this realization, I renounced dieting forever. I decided that instead of trying to force myself to lose weight against my body's will, I would turn my attention toward understanding *why* my body wanted to be fat in the first place.

I then went on a quest for real answers. I spent hours a day learning everything I could about biochemistry, nutrition, neurobiology, and psychology. In the eighties, I attended The Warton School of Business at the University of Pennsylvania. While I was at Wharton, I became very interested in biochemistry and took a full curriculum of biology courses. I also did a year of research into cholesterol synthesis with Dr. Jose Rabinowitz at the VA medical hospital in Philadelphia. This gave me a solid enough background in biochemistry to make sense of all the current obesity research.

I plowed through twenty or thirty research reports a day, and after reading several hundred—if not a thousand—research reports, I rapidly became an expert in the most cutting-edge chemistry of obesity and weight loss. I also studied meditation, hypnosis, neuro-linguistic programming, psycho-linguistics, Thought Field Therapy, Tai Chi, Chi Kung, and the field of consciousness research. I even studied quantum physics. I was convinced that the answers lay somewhere between the space that separates the mind from the body.

But more than anything, I started studying my own body. I stopped seeing it as the enemy that just wouldn't listen to me. I realized my problem was not my body but my lack of understanding how to operate it. From that moment on, I started listening to my body very closely. I also stopped trying to push it around and force it to do something against its will. Instead, I became its student, and as a result, I started learning from my body.

Because I became a receptive student, my body became a highly effective teacher. It taught me why it wanted to be fat and what I would have to do to make it want to be thin.

As soon as I understood that there were reasons why my body wanted to be fat, I stopped dieting. What was the point of trying to diet if it was not going to solve the problem? I later discovered that not only does dieting not work, but if your body already *wants* to be fat, dieting will only make it want to be fatter.

Giving up dieting forever was the greatest and most liberating thing I had ever done.

I hated dieting.

I hated being so obsessed with food and treating every hunger signal as a battle I had to fight. I hated ranking every day according to how good I had been: "Oh, I was good today!" Or on a bad day: "Okay, today's a baddy, so let's just go for it. Let's go to the store and buy every cake, cookie, brownie, and flavor of ice cream. No, don't get chocolate! It has too many calories. Get this one that's fat-free—the vanilla bean ice-latte sorbet-banana-sunshine. And now that you're here, you might as well try the passion fruit and the peach as well. Ah, screw it! Since you're getting all that, you might as well get the double fudge, chocolate brownie, *real* ice cream. But don't just get that one, because today's *the day*; if you're going to do it, you might as well try that other one you've been hankering for too."

Dieting and binging had been my way of life, but after my realization, I gave all that up. I let it go and I stopped having good days and bad days; I stopped treating every hunger pang as a battle. If I was hungry, I would eat, and if I wasn't hungry, I wouldn't eat. If I wanted the double-fudge whatever, I'd have some. I had a bite, or two, or ten, or the whole thing. Because I was no longer counting, I didn't care. I also realized that a lot of other people don't count what they eat. They pay no attention to what they're eating and yet they never gain a pound. I call these people the "naturally thin."

Naturally thin people have no dysfunctional relationships with food. They have no good days and no bad days. They don't have foods they can't have. They eat whatever they want, whenever they want. They don't agonize about what's best for them. They just don't care. They simply eat when they're hungry and that's that—end of story.

So I started living that way. I started living like a naturally thin person, eating whatever I wanted, whenever I wanted, but with one difference: I made sure I added certain foods that I knew had the nutrients my body needed in a form that I could digest and assimilate.

In the beginning, the foods I craved were still the same. I was still eating a lot of junk food as a rebound effect from having denied myself so many things for so long. However, that gradually changed, and I started craving not only less food but also much healthier foods. Nowadays, if my body's hungry, it's hungry for a reason. I respect that and I don't judge it. I just listen to it and do my best to obey. The types of foods my body now craves are fresh live fruits and rich colorful salads. Food that I had once seen as a chore or a punishment to eat now tastes richer to me than anything I had in my fifteen years of overindulgence and excessive living in New York.

My tastes have been completely transformed. Most of what I used to crave was not really food. It was nothing but sugar and artificial flavors. There was almost nothing I was putting into my body except empty calories. So, in actuality, one of the reasons I was hungry all the time was that I was *starving for nutrients.*

I was starving my body. Since it couldn't use the food I was eating, it just stayed hungry and continued to starve. No matter how much I ate, my body wasn't getting nourishment because there was nothing in the food I was eating to nourish it. Imagine feeding a baby nothing but soda. That's what comes to mind when I think of that period in my life.

The baby needed mother's milk and I was giving it cola. So what choice did it have but to keep crying? It had to do *something*. It had to ask for more of whatever I gave it—that was its only choice. Even though I weighed over 400 pounds and even though there were many days I ate over 5,000 calories, I was nonetheless starving *nutritionally*.

My body was in perpetual starvation mode despite a seemingly infinite supply of nutritionally depleted food, and despite carrying around enough excess reserve food in the form of fat to last the next three lifetimes.

And it wasn't just my body that was starving. I was starving in every aspect of my life. I was starving mentally, emotionally, and spiritually. I was not listening to or following my heart. I was living according to a preconceived notion of what my life was supposed to be. My heart was telling me to go in a different direction altogether, and I wasn't listening. Instead, I found myself constantly trying to protect myself from all the changes my heart was calling me to make. As a result, I was starving at a soul level—starving for the experiences that my soul wanted to have in this life.

I was spending all my time working indoors in New York City when I wanted to be out in the fresh, unspoiled wilderness. I was stuck in an office, nine to five, five days a week, and for the lion's share of the day, I was looking at fluorescent light, smelling industrial carpet, and hearing the same beeps, rings, and sales pitches that I had been hearing every day for fifteen years. I was not just starving for nutrients—I was starving for life.

In my heart of hearts, I wanted to be somewhere else.

But what could I do? I was making two or three times more as a bond trader than at anything else I could have done. What's more, I needed the money because I had three mortgages, two car leases, and thirteen credit cards that were nearly maxed-out. I was locked in the office, and chained to my commitments and financial obligations with what we in the business call the "golden handcuffs." I was locked into my life, and I was not getting out any time soon.

But as I started listening closely to my body, I was finally able to hear my heart. For the first time, I could hear my heart telling me I was suffocating. But because I had no plan in mind, all I could do was listen and dream.

Even though I did not have the courage or the strength to change my life, it was destined to change dramatically.

A month after my realization, I was supposed to fly to San Francisco for what had the potential to be one of the most important business meetings of my life. I was to meet with a major brokerage company to discuss with them the prospect of buying the business I had built. It was a day that could change my life forever. This meeting had the potential to make all my dreams come true.

Anytime I flew to San Francisco I always chose a non-stop flight from Newark Airport. However, on this particular occasion, my business partner chose to save one hundred and fifty dollars, and booked me on a cheaper but much more inconvenient flight that was leaving in the afternoon from La Guardia Airport in New York. I didn't exactly relish the thought of having to negotiate two hours of traffic to get to La Guardia, spend three hundred dollars in parking, and endure a two-hour stopover in Cincinnati just to save one hundred and fifty dollars. Normally I would have done something about it, but something told me to just let it go, and so I did.

In the end, I never took that flight because the airport was closed on September 11, 2001, so I never flew to San Francisco for that business meeting. But the flight I originally wanted to take took off before the airports shut down. It was United Airlines Flight 93, already in the air by the time the first plane had crashed into the World Trade Center. The passengers on Flight 93 had time to hear about that. They had time to call their husbands and wives from their cell phones, to tell them how much they loved them and how much they meant to them, before they took charge of the situation and forced the highjackers to crash the plane onto a field in Pennsylvania. There were no survivors.

If I had taken Flight 93, I would have been leaving a 400-pound body behind, having spent my whole adult life in an office, being devitalized by and wilting under fluorescent lighting while hearing the same beeps, rings, and sales pitches.

That would have been my fate, but by the grace of God, I was given a second chance. Two weeks later, I arrived at my office, ready to have a great day, ready to really embrace my life and make the most of it—only to find out that my business was closed.

The brokerage company that kept all our accounts had gone under as part of the stock market backlash after 9/11. They had lost eighty million dollars overnight. As a result, our assets and our clients' assets had all been frozen. Not a single client could transfer any money out of his or her account or make any trades for three weeks. The second that they could take their money out, they did. That was the end of my business.

The company I struggled so hard to create—all the sacrifices, fights, and challenges—had vanished in an instant. I sat at my desk in a stupor. Unable to do anything else, I stared blankly at my computer screen until it suddenly dawned on me.

My life had been spared again.

At that moment, I felt an overwhelming desire to make my *real* dreams come true, so I did the one thing that was in my heart of hearts to do. I purchased two one-way tickets to Western Australia for my wife and myself. This had been our dream for a long time, and I was finally ready to start living it with nothing but faith and a desire to follow my heart.

That night I came home with two big pieces of news for my wife. One was that I was out of business, and the other was that we were moving to Australia in six month's time. Two weeks later, she had news for me. We were expecting our first child.

Six months later, we were on a plane to Australia. We had no idea what we were going to do for the rest of our lives, and we didn't care. I had faith that I was being guided and that, as long as I was following my heart, I would be on the path on which I was meant to be. To this day, I still listen to my heart and follow its guidance.

For me, transforming my body was to a very large extent about transforming my life. But there were other issues I needed to address. I was under extreme stress, and as you'll learn later, certain types of stress can trick your body into wanting to be fat and activate what I call the "FAT Programs." I also had a condition that I call "emotional obesity," which occurs when someone actually feels safer being fat. I had to deal with a lot of different issues.

In the following pages, I'll discuss the many different reasons why our bodies want to be fat. Most of you reading this book will only have one or two issues that you will need to focus on. You just have to understand them, and then learn how to address and eliminate them. The whole process can be very easy, and after reading this book, you'll know exactly what to do.

But for now, the only thing you need to understand is that if you have more than about 10 pounds to lose and you can't lose them, it's because your body has a reason why it's holding on to extra weight. Your body wants to be fat, and as long as this is the case, fighting it just won't work.

Your body is holding all the cards. It controls your appetite. If it wants to, it can make you crave all the wrong foods in insatiable amounts. It controls your metabolism, so even if you think you can control how much food you put in your body, it controls how much energy it will burn and how much it will store. Your body can make you so tired all the time that you have no energy to exercise, even if you have just hired the fitness trainer to the stars.

Your body also has the final say on what it will do with whatever food you put into it. It can choose to store as much of it in your fat cells as it wants to. It can choose storage in your fat cells over providing energy to your muscles. In addition, when your body needs energy and you are not giving it enough food, it can burn muscle instead of fat.

Your body is the real boss. It controls all of your fat metabolism as well as many of your other basic survival functions in a tiny little area at the base of your brain—the "animal brain." This area determines how much sleep you need, how much air you need, and how fat or thin you should be. If you need more sleep, it will make you tired. If you need more oxygen, it will make you want to breathe harder. And if you need more fat, it will make you hungry. It's that simple. Try holding your breath long enough, and you soon realize that the urge to breathe is totally compelling. And so it should be! Breathing is keeping you alive! Your body's fat storage mechanism works in exactly the same way. As long as your body is convinced that keeping you fat is keeping you safe, the urge to eat junk food will be equally compelling.

Fat people have always been accused of being weak, lazy, and overindulgent, not just by the general public but by the mainstream healthcare industry. I know every time I walked into a doctor's office I would get that oh-look-at-this-guy-that-doesn't-care-about-himself look. Nothing was further than the truth, but I'd get the look—EVERY TIME.

Imagine if someone said to you that your problem is you sleep too much and you should just sleep two hours a day. And everyone in society and in your life judged you for being weak and lazy because you slept so much. You could sleep two hours a night for a while, but sooner or later you'll need a big sleep—a "binge sleep"—because you're body is going to want it regardless of what society tells you.

IT'S EXACTLY THE SAME WITH FOOD.

You can cut your intake and force yourself to eat less for a while, but sooner or later you're going to need a big "binge eat." That's because your body is forcing you to eat more in order to keep you at a certain weight.

One of the things I've been crusading for is an official apology from the medical community for endorsing the common stereotypes that fat people lack self-discipline. Fortunately, I've noticed that the situation is improving. There are now many enlightened doctors and healthcare professionals who understand the real reason that so many people are obese, but we still have a long way to go. Conventional medical wisdom still says that weight loss is simply a matter of calories in and calories out, and that fat people should "just eat less." To those who feel that way, I say, "just breathe less" or "just sleep less." Only after truly thinking about the impossibility of those commands will they know exactly what it's like to struggle with obesity.

There's no way anyone, doctor or otherwise, can ever possibly imagine what it's like to be in a body that's forcing you to be fat and to eat too much, unless they have lived through it. That being said, the most cutting-edge research now confirms that losing weight is not just about "calories in and calories out," and that it hasn't got anything to do with "discipline." Dr. Jeffrey M. Friedman, the "father of fat," discoverer of the hormone leptin, and, without question, the most important and knowledgeable expert on obesity of the twenty-first century, says that we have to stop blaming fat people and that "obesity cannot be ascribed to a breakdown in will power."[1]

Thank you, Dr. Friedman! Please spread the word.

So, the first step is to understand that it's not about will power and to come to terms with this. Rather than struggle in vain against overwhelming "animal brain" instincts to keep you alive, all you need to do is understand why your body wants to be fat and then eliminate those reasons. Eliminate the reasons your body wants to be fat and it will want to be thin—naturally.

The truth is your body doesn't want to be fat in order to hurt you or punish you. The only reason your body is fat right now is because, for some reason, it thinks it is in your best interest to be fat. But as soon as you identify the problems and you start addressing them, everything changes.

You'll be able to tell immediately when your body no longer wants to be fat. You won't be as hungry and you won't think about food as much. You'll have more energy and enthusiasm, and you'll no longer be at war with your body.

It may not show on the outside right away, but you'll know immediately that something has changed on the inside. Your relationship to food will change, and your relationship to your body will change. Your body won't be undermining your efforts anymore.

Once you remove the reasons why your body wants to be fat, your relationship to exercise will also change. Right now you may think you hate to exercise; I don't blame you. There is a very real reason why you hate exercise: your body doesn't want you to exercise since exercising will make you lose weight. As long as your body wants to be fat, it won't want you to be active and burning calories, because that will only make keeping the weight harder for it.

Your body makes you tired and lethargic so that even the thought of exercise causes you pain. This is not a coincidence; this is something your body is doing intentionally so that you will remain sedentary.

However, once you remove the reasons why your body thinks it needs to be fat, it will want to be active again. Exercise will no longer be a chore, and being active may even become one of your greatest joys.

I repeat, although it may not show right away, it is only a matter of time before you'll lose all the weight. You'll know that the change will have already happened on the inside, and it's only a matter of time before everyone else is going see it on the outside.

I knew over two years before anyone else did what was going on inside my body. I didn't talk about it much, but I knew what was going on. I might have been walking around in a 400-pound body, but in my mind's eye, I held the image of a teenager who weighed 180 pounds. From that moment on, it was a certainty.

The most amazing thing that happened to me was that the more I lost weight, the faster I lost it. I discovered there was a reason for this. Your body has complete control over how fast you burn fat. If it wants to be thinner, it will burn fat very quickly and easily. That's the biggest difference between my method and a diet: the thinner my body wanted to be, the faster I lost weight.

Diets all start out the same way. You lose weight very quickly at first, but then your weight loss slows down. Finally, you stop losing weight altogether only to gain it back a short time later.

I didn't lose weight quickly at first; I lost it *slowly*. I lost about 25 pounds over the first six months. That's around a pound a week. For someone who weighed over 400 pounds that wasn't setting any record.

But then, instead of slowing down, I started losing weight faster. I lost another 150 pounds at a rate of 2 pounds a week, and I lost 20 more at a rate of 3 pounds a week.

I lost the last 20 pounds—the weight that most people say is impossible to lose—at a rate of *5 pounds a week*. A rate that was *five times faster* than the first 20 pounds. Not only were those last few pounds possible to lose, they actually flew off me. My body simply couldn't stand to have an extra ounce of fat on it. It shed every ounce of those last remaining pounds. I could see all of my stomach muscles again, which was something I had dreamed of doing but hadn't been able to do since I was a kid.

What's more, I showed almost no signs of ever having been morbidly obese. My skin became tight and firm. This fact continues to astound doctors and laypeople alike.

I didn't have to do much to make this happen and neither will you. It simply wasn't a struggle. There are really only three things that I did from day one:

1. I never let a day go by without making sure I had given my body the nourishment it needed in a form that it could digest and assimilate. The focus was on adding what was missing.

2. I spent at least some time every day practicing techniques I developed to address the mental and emotional causes of obesity.

3. Every night, as I was going to sleep, I visualized my ideal body exactly the way I wanted it to look and feel. Eventually that vision became a reality.

I also used visualization in many other ways. For example, in May of 2003 I entered a twelve-week weight-loss challenge. By then I had already lost over 110 pounds and I figured, since I was already losing weight so quickly, I might as well enter a competition. I wanted something to help accelerate my weight loss, so I developed a visualization technique to kill my sugar cravings.

I didn't actually win the competition, but the visualization technique proved to be extremely effective. I have continued to use that visualization technique, and I simply never crave sugar anymore.

Everything else pretty much happened on its own.

Did I start eating less? Of course I did! But that was because I just wasn't as hungry. Did I start eating healthier? Definitely! But that's just because I started craving healthier foods. Did I exercise? You bet I did! And I enjoyed every minute of it. It's what my body wanted me to do. But don't worry; in this book, I will never ask you to force yourself to exercise or force yourself to do anything.

I will only ask you to do three things:

1. Never go a single day without adding the nutrients your body is starving for.
2. Listen to my evening visualization CD[2] or spend at least ten minutes a day practicing the visualization techniques I talk about in this book.
3. Listen to your heart and to your body.

If you're willing to do these three things, I would like to invite you to join me on what may be one of the most satisfying journeys of your life, with the potential to not only transform your body but to transform any aspect of your life that you desire.

—Jon Gabriel

NOTES

1. See J. Bonner, "Jeffrey Friedman, Discoverer of Leptin, Receives Gairdner Passano Award," The Rockefeller University Office of Communications and Public Affairs Website (April 13, 2005): http://runews.rockefeller.edu/index.php?page=engine&id=178.

2. Please go to http://www.gabrielmethod.com/cd for instructions on how to download *The Gabriel Method Evening Visualization* CD for free.

PART I

The Principles

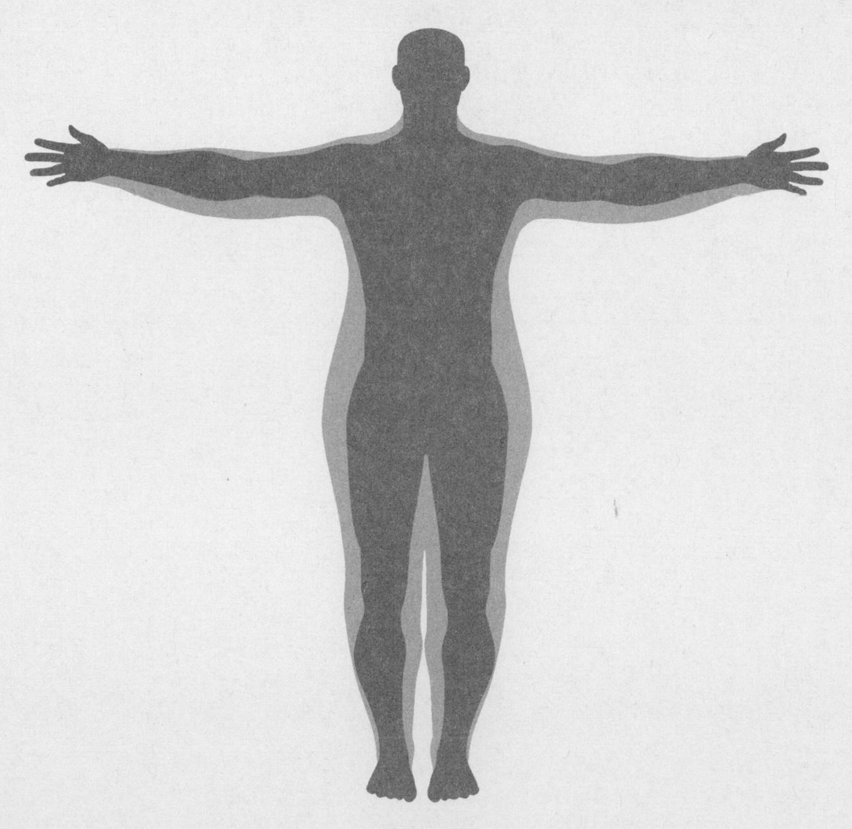

1

The FAT Programs: The Real Reason You're Fat

Let's get this out of the way: You're not fat because you eat too much! You're not weak or lazy or overindulgent or undisciplined or any of the typical "fat" stereotypes that are both ignorant and reprehensible. You're fat because your body *wants* to be fat. This may sound ridiculous, I know, and it may even sound harsh. But as you'll see, this fact is actually very liberating because, once you understand why your body would want to be fat, the solution presents itself easily.

The first thing you have to understand is that your body has the ability to *force* you to gain weight—if, for whatever reason, it wants to be fat—in the same way that your body has the ability to force you to breathe. Your body has certain genetic survival programs built into it that are designed to force you to either get fatter or hold on to fat whenever it feels that doing so will help keep you alive. I call these programs the FAT Programs. The FAT Programs are basically designed to turn your body into a fat storage machine.

FAT actually stands for "Famine And Temperature." In our distant past, it was advantageous for these programs to be on. During famines and ice ages, having excess fat on your body helped keep you alive, so a fat storage survival mechanism came into play. Pregnant women also have their FAT Programs turned on in order to cause them to gain the necessary body weight they need to nurture a growing fetus.[1] These programs are common to all mammals. Hibernating animals, for example, have their FAT Programs turned on in the months prior to winter in order to force them to gain as much weight as possible.[2]

Even though today most of us no longer have things like famines to worry about, these FAT Programs are still very much a part of our genetic inheritance. The problem is that sometimes your body can be tricked into activating these programs, so your confused body thinks that being fat or staying fat is, for some reason, protecting you. Your body is actually acting in your best interest. It's not trying to punish you and it doesn't hate you.

When the FAT Programs are on, certain subtle hormonal and chemical changes take place in your body that will virtually ensure that you get fat and stay fat.

This is what happens:

Chemical changes cause:	And the result is that:
You to be hungrier and crave more fattening foods.	You consume more calories.
Your metabolism to slow down; you become tired, lethargic, and sedentary.	You burn fewer calories.
Your body to go into perpetual fat storage mode. It becomes very efficient at storing fat and resists burning it.	All the excess calories you are consuming get stored in your fat cells and don't come out.

With these chemical and hormonal changes taking place, your body directs you to be hungry, have more cravings, and consume more calories while at the same time burning fewer calories and storing all it can in your fat cells. Right now, this is what you are experiencing and this is why you are fat. For some reason, your body has been tricked into activating the FAT Programs. It *could* happen to anyone and it *would* happen to anyone under the same circumstances. So please let go of any guilt, frustration, or other negative feelings you might be experiencing about not being able to lose weight. There is nothing wrong with you! Your FAT Programs are on, that's all. You are not any "weaker" or "less disciplined" than thin people.

The only difference between you and those naturally thin people is that your FAT Programs are turned on and theirs are not. That is it. If anything, you are probably stronger and more disciplined than thin people. Naturally thin people eat whatever they want. Where is the discipline in that? You, at least, make an effort to control yourself. The sad irony of the situation is that all your efforts to control yourself, although well intentioned, may not only be exacerbating the problem, they may even be the cause of it!

As I am sure you must know by now, struggle doesn't work. If it did, there would have been no need to buy this book at all. What works is to get your body to *want* to be thin. When your body wants to be thin, the FAT Programs are turned off, you quickly and easily lose weight, and you keep it off without struggle and without dieting.

Understanding Why Your Body Would Want to Be Fat

Here's the only concept you need to get in this whole book. Once you get this, everything else just falls into place.

Your body wants to be fat anytime it decides that being fat is the best way to keep you safe.

As far as your body is concerned, life is all about safety. Your body is not your enemy and it is not out to get you; it's just trying to protect you. Actually, your body has a brilliant logic that makes perfect sense. All you have to do is understand your body's logic and work with it as opposed to struggling against it. You have to convince your body, using its language and its reasoning, that being thin is the best way to keep you safe.

Once your body understands that being thin is the best way to keep you safe, your body will *want* to be thin and the weight will fall off.

The connection between being fat and being safe may seem odd, but it's true. In today's world, there is absolutely nothing about being fat that will make you safer. But your body doesn't understand today's world. Your body is programmed to protect you from the threats and uncertainties of a prehistoric world, where daily survival threats came down to three things—starving, freezing, and being eaten.

For countless generations, our ancestors had to worry about these three threats. As a result, our bodies are now brilliantly designed to protect us against them. Today, however, most of us no longer have to worry about starving, freezing, or being eaten. These are not the threats of our modern day world, but our bodies don't know this. Our bodies still function based on the same genetic programming that has protected us since the dawn of time.

So how did gathering and storing fat protect you against these ancient survival threats? If you were living in an environment where there was never enough food and you did not know when your next meal would be, having excess fat on your body would help keep you alive. The more fat you had on your body, the longer you could survive. In the same way, if you were living in a cold climate or during a long, harsh winter without the benefit of houses and central heating, having excess fat would also act as insulation. Fat protects your vital organs and your extremities from the cold.

So in the case of famine and cold weather, your body would want to be fat because, under these conditions, being fat can keep you alive.

However, being fat does not always keep you safe. It can also put you at risk of being eaten. If you were living in a land where there were man-eating predators, fat would no longer be your friend. Fat becomes your enemy. Because the fatter you are, the slower you are. This means if something is chasing you, the chances of escaping are slimmer. In these circumstances, your body would want to be thin because being thin is the best way to keep you fast and therefore safe. In this case, being thin could save your life.

In each of these examples, your chances of surviving are very much dependent on how fat or thin you are. Most living environments in our past had some combination of the big three threats—starving, freezing, and being eaten—and it was up to your body to decide the perfect weight that would make you the safest in any given scenario. You did not want to be so thin that you could not survive until your next meal, and you did not want to be so fat that you could not escape an attack.

This is where our body's brilliant logic was essential. Our bodies could quickly determine how much fat would be the ideal amount for us to carry around in any living condition, adjusting this "ideal weight" as situations changed. Our body's brilliant adaptability is the reason we are here today. This amazing flexibility protected our ancestors successfully from threats since the dawn of time. For this, we should be eternally grateful.

Unfortunately, this is all irrelevant today. In today's world of excess, fat doesn't make us any safer in the least, as I'm sure you consciously know. But our bodies don't know this. They still have the same genetic programming.

The problem is that the stresses of modern day life produce chemical signals in our bodies and brains. Sometimes those chemical signals are the *exact same chemical signals* that are produced when we are starving or freezing. If those chemical signals are the same as those produced when we are starving or freezing, our bodies will be "tricked" into thinking that we need to be fat in order to be safe, causing our bodies to activate the FAT Programs. This is what is happening to you. The stresses and struggles of modern day life are tricking your body into activating your FAT Programs.

In a sense, when you try to force yourself to lose weight while these programs are operating, you're violating your body's natural laws. Your body is trying to make you fatter and you are trying to make it thinner. That, to me, is the definition of struggle—a struggle your body will always win because of the power of this hard-wired program.

The way to lose weight is not to struggle or fight against your body. The way to lose weight is to figure out what's turning your FAT Programs on and getting your body to turn them off.

If you are currently carrying extra weight, then your body believes it is not safe to lose weight; it is fighting for your life. When your body believes that it is safe to lose weight—or better, safer to be thin—your body will *force* you to lose weight. You will be working with your body's natural laws instead of violating them. Weight loss will then become automatic, effortless, and inevitable.[3]

NOTES

1. See D. R. Grattan and S. R. Ladyman, "Region-Specific Reduction in Leptin-Induced Phosphorylation of Signal Transducer and Activator of Transcription-3 (sTAT3) in the Rat Hypothalamus Is Associated with Leptin Resistance During Pregnancy," *Endocrinology* 145, no. 8 (2004): 3704–3711.

2. See A. Tups, C. Adam, C. Ellis, K. Moar, J. Mercer, M. Klingenspor, and T. Logie, "Photoperiodic Regulation of Leptin Sensitivity in the Siberian Hamster, *Phodopus sungorus*, Is Reflected in Arcuate Nucleus SOCS-3 (Suppressor of Cytokine Signaling) Gene Expression," *Endocrinology* 145, no. 3 (2004): 1185–1193.

3. If you are scientifically minded and want to know the specific hormones that regulate the FAT Programs, see the appendix (page 185).

2

Jessie's Law

There are two levels at which you can look at weight loss, and most people are looking at the first level, the level of your metabolism—calories in, calories out, diets, pills, surgery, fat burning secrets, behavior modification, the whole endless list that fills book stores and libraries. All these ideas operate on the same premise: that you somehow have to drug, cut open, discipline, control, fight, or otherwise force your body to lose weight. That's where all the research is, and that's what everyone's focused on.

But as you now know, there's a higher and much more relevant level to weight loss, and that is the level of your body's "ideal weight"—how fat or thin your body *desires* to be. The problem is that the things that force your body to lose weight are not the same things that get your body to want to be thin. In fact, they usually have the exact opposite effect.

So if you want to lose weight easily and sustainably, and be done with diets and discipline forever, you simply have to get your body to want to be thin. To illustrate how this works in real life, let's look at the story of Jessie and how his experience contributed to forming what I call "Jessie's Law."

Jessie

Jessie's understanding of metabolism and calorie control were nonexistent. Jessie had never even been to school, so he couldn't read or write, and while he was quite smart for a housecat, he wasn't exactly a rocket scientist either. Just entering his young adulthood, Jessie was what you could describe as pleasantly plump. He didn't work all that hard and spent most of his spare time loafing around the house, just like other cats.

Buddy, our next-door neighbors' 120-pound mastiff, hated cats. Every afternoon, Jessie took a pleasant stroll over to our neighbors' yard and would lay on the grass to tease poor Buddy, who was locked indoors. Jessie would mosey on over, lie down on the grass, yawn, and stretch, and Buddy would go crazy, barking and screaming from inside the house.

One day, the neighbors got sick of it and let Buddy out. Buddy shot out of his yard like a freight train firing on all pistons. I never saw anything so big move so fast. He and Jessie ran off into the woods, and I didn't see Jessie for the rest of the day.

The next day, Jessie came back limping. Buddy had gotten a hold of Jessie's leg and bit it. I nursed Jessie back to health and he was fine, but then something amazing happened. Over the next few weeks, he got very thin and wiry. People started commenting on his weight drop, and they suggested that a vet check him for worms. But I knew exactly why Jessie had become so thin. Jessie's body wanted to be thinner to keep him alive. A new stress had come into his life, and Jessie was adapting to the stress.

Let's look at it from Jessie's perspective:

Stress—Big Mean Dog
Interpretation—If Big Mean Dog gets me, I will die.
Reaction—Run for my life.
Adaptation—Get thinner and faster so next time this literal son-of-a-bitch tries to catch me, I'll outrun him and I'LL BE SAFE.

The important part of this equation is the adaptation strategy, and it was the adaptation that made Jessie's body *want* to be thinner.

That's a question you may want to ask yourself right now: "How is my body adapting to the stresses in my life?"

But there's more to this story.

As a result of his adaptation, Jessie stayed lean and lanky—too thin in fact, by my estimation. Even though I started feeding him an all-you-can-eat diet of rich, canned cat food, chicken, and fish, he wasn't putting on any weight. His body got the urgent message that being thin equals being safe, and all of the sudden he had the metabolism of a greyhound.

I knew that no matter how much food I gave Jessie he wasn't going to gain any weight. In fact, as long as his body knew that food was limitless, his body would have no need to store fat. The land of excess he was living in just didn't make his body want to be any fatter.

So I decided to do something about it. I put him on a diet. That's right, I put him on a diet because I knew from experience that the best way to get your body to want to be fatter is to diet. Rather than give him an all-you-can-eat buffet of scrumptious foods, I fed him sparingly, only once a day, despite all of his protests. I made sure that I gave him what he needed, but there was no excess. I did this for a month, and in the last week, I only fed him dry food, something that he was definitely not accustomed to. You may think that this sounds cruel, but this is exactly what we do to ourselves all the time when we go on a diet.

After a month of this minimalist fare, I went back to giving him an all-you-can-eat buffet of all his favorite foods, and sure enough, he gained weight. I basically turned on his Fat Programs. That's what dieting does. And this is exactly why diets don't work: they trick your body into thinking you're living in a time of famine and make your body want to be fatter.

Let's face it: if diets worked there'd be one diet (maybe two), everyone would go on it, everyone would lose weight, and that would be the end of it. There wouldn't be thousands of diets out there and hundreds of new ones coming out every year, all operating on the same premise that you can somehow force yourself to lose weight. If diets worked, the issue would be done. No one would be talking about it anymore. The reason everyone's talking about it is because the very premise is flawed, and every approach founded on that same premise is, unfortunately, doomed to the same fate.

Jessie never went back to his pleasantly plump days. He stayed somewhere in the middle. The two opposing stresses balanced each other out. Buddy kept turning off his Fat Programs, and I kept turning them back on. His body settled on an ideal weight so he was not too fat to run away from Buddy and not too thin to survive my next artificial famine. (Sorry, Jessie. It was all in the name of science. Anyway, girl cats don't like guys who are too skinny. They want a mate with a little meat on his bones.)

Applying Jessie's Law in the Real World

Today most of us don't have to worry about dogs or tigers chasing us, or famines, but we have other stresses, such as nutritional famines, toxins, radiation, noise pollution, war, crime, mortgages, stock market fluctuations, savings and loan scandals, commuter traffic, rude customers, sick relatives, unemployment, not getting enough dates, getting too many dates, abusive partners, abusive family members, abusive bosses, abusive clients—the list goes on and on. And all of these stresses can trigger chemical reactions in our bodies that trick our animal brain into activating the FAT Programs.

There are many reasons why your body can be deceived into activating your FAT Programs, and here's a list of the most common ones:

Chronic Yo-Yo Dieting: If you're constantly forcing yourself to eat less or denying yourself the foods that you're craving, then you're also causing your body to think that food is limited, that you are living in a time of famine, or both. Dieting is the act of forcibly trying to control either the quantity or quality of what you are eating. Any type of dieting is a form of starvation. This type of starvation can make your body think that it needs to carry around extra fat and, therefore, activate the FAT Programs.

Nutritional Starvation: You may be eating to your heart's content, but your body may still be starving *nutritionally*.

This can happen in four main ways:

- Certain essential nutrients are missing from your diet.
- The nutrients in your food have been destroyed.
- You are not digesting your food properly.
- Your cells aren't absorbing the nutrients.

Toxins: Your body is using fat to help protect you from toxins, which are stored in your fat cells. In the same way that your body used to use fat to protect you from the cold, it is also using fat to help insulate and protect your vital organs from the poisons in your food and your environment.

Radiation: Fat also absorbs radiation, and your body uses fat to insulate and protect your vital organs from radiation.

Medication: Certain medications can artificially activate the FAT Programs. For further specific details on potentially problematic medications, see page 118.

Food Additives: Processed foods, artificial sweeteners, and flavor enhancers are radically different from the foods our ancestors ate. Our bodies don't know how to digest them. They can cause a kind of hormonal chaos that turns on the FAT Programs. I am not saying that you should avoid them or any foods that you are craving, because that would be a diet and diets don't work. On the other hand, the Gabriel Method increases your body's desire for real foods and allows any cravings that you might have for these "fake" foods to fall away by themselves—without dieting, without struggle, and without a futile and superhuman use of will power. When your body wants to be thin, you'll simply no longer crave foods that make it fat.

Mental and Emotional Threats: Your body treats all mental and emotional stresses as if they are *literal physical threats*. Every time you feel stress, you are sending a chemical message to your body, and that message is: "I am not safe. Do something!" Your body is programmed to do whatever it can to protect you, but the only types of threats your body understands are physical threats, not emotional ones. So when you are upset emotionally, your body actually thinks you are in danger *physically*.

To your body, "threat" means that either something is attacking you, or that you are possibly starving or freezing to death. Mental and emotional threats can sometimes produce the same chemical signals in your body that starving and freezing produce. When this happens, your body gets confused into thinking that you need to be fat in order to be safe, thus activating the FAT Programs.

Here are some examples of mental and emotional threats that can confuse your body into thinking that being fat can help keep you safe:

Mental Starvation: Your body only understands one form of starvation and that is *physical* starvation, but you can also be starving in a mental or emotional sense. For example, you can be starving for love, fun, joy, intimacy, life experiences, or a deeper spiritual connection. All of these mental and emotional longings can cause the same chemical signals in your brain that physical starvation causes. These signals can all activate the FAT Programs.

Fear of Scarcity: The fear of not having enough money or of losing something you value can send a message to your body that resources are limited, but the only resource your body understands is food. As far as your body is concerned, it's the only thing you can save. Any fear that resources may become limited is interpreted as fear of famine. If the body thinks a famine is coming, it will want to stock up on as much fat as possible.

Emotional Obesity: You may not be aware of it consciously, but if at some level you have made the association that being fat makes you feel safer, or that it is in some way serving an emotional need, you have "emotional obesity." This is one of those instances where your body is getting it right. In this case, your body really is protecting you; it is making you feel safer emotionally.

Dysfunctional Beliefs: Beliefs have a much greater control over our physical bodies than we give them credit for. There are hundreds of documented examples of terminally ill individuals who believed that they would be healed and then were. There are also examples of people who believed they would get sick and then became ill. There are even examples of people who believed that they were going to die, and for no other reason, they died.

In the same way, negative and dysfunctional beliefs surrounding obesity and weight loss can activate the FAT Programs. If you believe you were meant to be fat, born to be fat, or deserve to be fat, or if you believe that losing weight is difficult or impossible, then your body gets fat or stays fat simply because that's your belief. It is understandable why you may have arrived at some of these incorrect conclusions, but that's only because you've been approaching weight loss in the wrong way—from the outside in, by forcing yourself to eat less and denying yourself the foods that you're craving. Weight loss is easy and effortless when you get your body to *want* to be thin. In order to do this, however, one of the things you have to do is eliminate the dysfunctional beliefs that are getting in your way.

Understanding what triggers the FAT Programs and how to turn them off is really the key to everything. If you get this right, everything else is smooth sailing.

Envisioning Your End Result

When you have read and understood the tools in this book, my promise to you is that you can expect to:

- **Stop dieting:** You will never be asked to control your eating forcibly, neither the amount of food you are eating nor the type of foods you are craving. You can eat whatever you want whenever you want.
- **Nourish your body:** Rather than dieting, I'll ask you to add certain foods and to adopt positive eating habits. This

is designed to help nourish your body and remove starvation in its various forms. This will also reduce the level of toxins entering your body. By taking this approach, you will be eliminating the physical signals that are activating the FAT Programs. Therefore, even though you are not dieting, you will be less hungry and will naturally start to crave healthier foods.

- **Eliminate the mental and emotional causes of obesity:** I'll show you simple, highly effective techniques for eliminating the mental and emotional causes of obesity. These techniques involve two minutes of visualization at night, listening to my visualization CD, and/or practicing ten minutes of visualization during the day.

This is all you'll need to do to follow the approach that worked for me and Jessie, and for people all over the world, whether they know anything about diets or calories or not. The Gabriel Method simply and systematically eliminates all the conceivable physical, mental, and emotional factors that are causing your body to activate the FAT Programs.

If you are willing to do this, I invite you to embark on a journey with me that will put an end to the struggle once and for all. Our journey has the potential to transform not only your body but also your entire life.

So let's start by looking in greater depth at some of the mental and emotional stresses that can cause your body to activate the FAT Programs, and what you can do to eliminate them. Don't worry if it seems like a lot of information. In the final section, I'll incorporate everything into a simple, step-by-step approach.

PART II

Nonphysical Stresses that Activate the FAT Programs

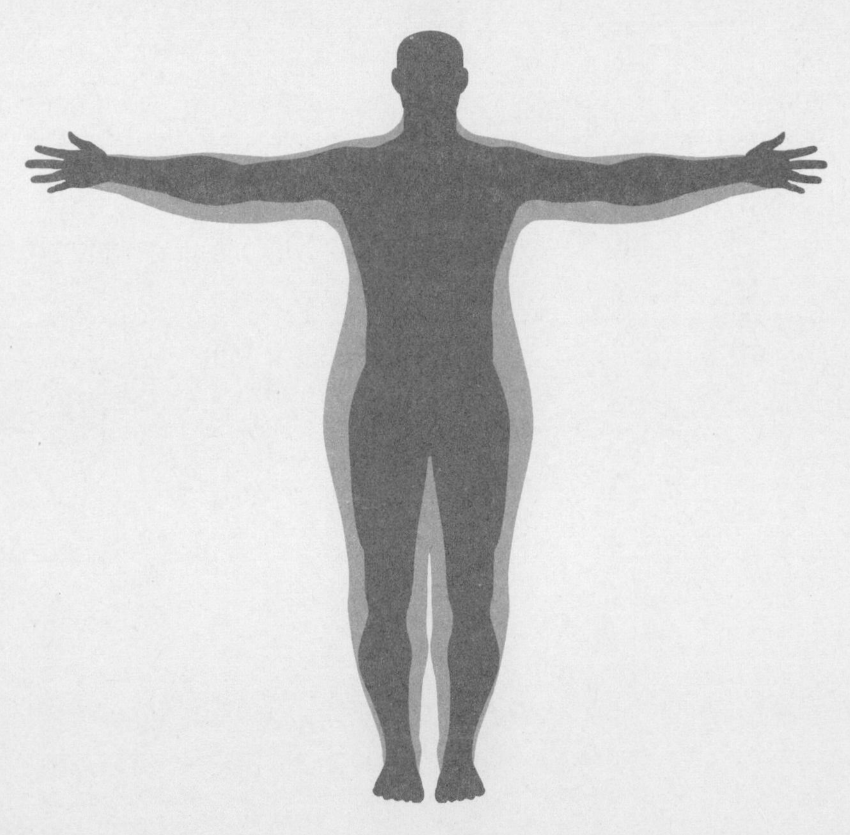

3

Mental Causes of Obesity

Most weight-loss programs place minimal attention on the mind–body connection, and this is where they fall short. Nothing is more important than understanding the way the mind and body are communicating with each other, especially when it comes to stress.

This is why feeling safe, and understanding and addressing mental and emotional stress is of paramount importance when you want to lose weight.

Keep in mind that when Jessie's body got the message "Thin = Safe," even giving him the richest, all-you-can-eat, optimal nutrition couldn't make him any fatter because his body didn't want to be fatter. No amount of raw calories could convince him of that. And when his body wanted to be fat because Fat = Safe, it was easy for him to put on weight.

Human lives tend to be more complicated than Jessie's, but not as far as our bodies are concerned. Every time you have mental or emotional stress, it generates chemical changes in your body—chemistry that activates ancient survival programs inside us. But which program is it going to activate? Is it going to activate the "Buddy's chasing me" / thin program, or is it going to activate the famine program? Because if it activates the "Buddy program," it will make your body want to be thin, and if it activates the famine program, it will make your body want to be fat.

This explains why the same superficial stress makes some people put on weight and some people lose it. In an abusive, emotional situation, one person may put on weight as a shield, while another person will shed weight in preparation for running away. It's all very primal. It's all a result of basic instincts. And it's these basic instincts that have kept your body locked into an unacceptable weight situation. But the facts also provide your key to liberation.

If you don't address this point of mental and emotional fat-causing stress, any type of eating or behavior modification you make will yield marginal results at best. Not only that, it will be exhausting and extremely frustrating. It will feel like you're driving a car with the emergency break on.

But when you do get this point right and feel safe, and your body is no longer interpreting the stresses in your life as a type of famine or harsh weather, your body will no longer want to be fat. Weight loss is not only easy, IT'S INEVITABLE. If your body wants to be thin, there is nothing you can do to stop it. Your metabolism will speed up, you will be less hungry, you will crave healthier foods, and you will become very efficient at burning fat.

So let's take a look at some of the most common forms of mental and emotional stress that may be activating your body's FAT Programs, and then examine what you can do to eliminate them:

Mental Starvation: Lack—The Modern Day Famine

It makes sense that our brains could interpret any mental or emotional stress that originates from a feeling of lack as a kind of starvation. In a sense, *any* lack is a form of starvation. Whether you feel that you don't have enough money, love, attention, or meaning in your life, the feeling is lack—not enough of something.

Our brain takes this message of lack and has to translate it into physical terms. The most crucial type of lack that the most primitive part of the brain understands is the physical lack of food, because food and water were the primary things our ancestors could be lacking. So, as a result, the brain can interpret any form of mental, emotional, or even spiritual lack as a lack of food.

The Daily Grind

What we commonly think of as stress—the frantic and sometimes desperate ongoing struggle to make ends meet and get ahead in life—can sometimes trick your body into thinking that it must be a time of famine, so it activates the FAT Programs.

This chronic stress can very easily mimic the chemical signals that are created when we are starving; chronic stress is alarming but not immediately life threatening. It's not like a tiger chasing you, for example, so running away won't necessarily make it better. It's more like a famine or a cold winter: it's always there and you just have to take it—grin and bear it.

Interestingly, famine and the daily grind have something in common. Your body perceives them both as chronic, low-level threats to your long-term survival. When you don't eat enough every day, day in and day out, you're not going to drop dead on any one day from starvation. But over time, if left unchecked, you could starve to death.

In the same way, in the modern day famine, if you're late for work on any given day, nothing is going to happen. If you're late every day, day after day, you might get fired. If you get fired, you might not be able to make ends meet. If you can't make ends meet, you might not be able to afford your house or apartment, or even have enough money for food. If you don't have enough money for food, you might starve. In a sense, your brain is correct in interpreting this fear as a fear of starvation.

Fear of job loss or worrying about making ends meet does not automatically make every person fat. Every individual reacts differently to stress. But the truth of the matter is you are more likely to gain weight the more worried you are about losing your job or about making ends meet. Studies have shown that people in particularly stressful working environments and families with less money are more likely to be fat.[1]

However, you can be a millionaire and still be worried about making ends meet, or about getting ahead. It's how much you worry about it and how your brain interprets the fear that matters, not the objective reality of the situation.

Spiritual Starvation

Spiritual longing is really a desire to connect with our soul, our creator, or whatever else we may chose to call our one true source. This can be a type of starvation that activates the Fat Programs, but there's more to it than that. When we feel disconnected, food can sometimes be a way of connecting with the outside world. Think about what you're doing when you're eating—you are taking something that is outside of you and you are bringing it inside you in a very intimate way. You are connecting and merging with that food, and that food becomes you; eating becomes a surrogate for the true connection that we desire. When we have spiritual starvation, there can be the tendency to "fill the soul" by eating.

You can also be starving for meaning and purpose in your life, and this can activate the FAT Programs. As a matter of fact, researchers have discovered a statistical correlation between lives lived with a sense of purpose and a healthier weight.[2] Living life in a way that we feel is meaningful—feeling like there is a purpose to our existence—nourishes our soul. Meaning and purpose are "soul food," and many of us are starving for this essential, nonphysical nutrient.

What Are You "Weighting" For?—Follow Your Heart

Here's a bit of practical (or impractical, depending on the situation) advice. Whatever you really want to do but are afraid to do—DO IT. Take the chance—follow your heart. It's essential to listen to the messages from your heart. These messages are your soul's desire. They communicate to you what you are meant to be doing at any given time in your life. If you don't follow these messages, you will inevitably be straying from your life's path.

If you don't listen to the messages from your heart, the feeling of longing and frustration is never going to go away; it will only get worse. Negativity constricts the flow of grace into your life, causing pain and emotional starvation.

I recently saw Gina, a friend of mine who I have not seen in several years. She wants to lose weight and is on a very austere, low-calorie, low-fat, low-carb diet. She's not even allowed sweet peppers because they have too many carbs.

Gina's a teacher, and she's tired of being a teacher. Exhausted, she says she would like to retire in a few years, but she doesn't have the money. In her spare time, she paints and has several hundred paintings in her shed to prove it. When she showed me the pictures in her portfolio, they took my breath away. She entered two of them in contests and won.

So I asked her the obvious question: Why aren't you selling your paintings? She said that she was not sure anyone would like them. And as she said this, she hunched her shoulders and tensed her muscles. You could tell Gina was uncomfortable with where the conversation was going.

I said to her, "Wait a minute! You're tired of what you're doing for a living, and your heart isn't in it. In the meantime, you *do* have something that you love doing, something you would do for free anyway and something you are obviously good at. You have already produced several hundred paintings that are just gathering dust. You would like to lose weight and you are starving yourself to try to do it. You would like to retire but you're not making enough money."

At that point I got a little animated, and I said, "Let me tell you something. Your weight problems, your financial problems, and most likely any other physical or mental pains you are experiencing all center on one single issue. You have something you love to do and were born to do, and you're turning your back on it. Having something that you love doing is a gift from the universe, and you're rejecting it. When you reject that kind of gift, you are rejecting the grace that goes along with it. As a result, you struggle, you yearn, and you starve." Then I told Gina in no uncertain terms: "Take the chance! Follow you heart!

Embrace your life's destiny!" When we said good-bye and Gina walked away, she looked shell-shocked. She was in a daze of realization.

This is a common theme. If we fail to follow our hearts, obesity is often the result. Yearning causes emotional starvation and activates the FAT Programs.

There's a simple rule to follow.

If you have something that you'd like to do, long to do, yearn to do but are afraid to do—take the chance. DON'T *WEIGHT*! FOLLOW YOUR HEART!

Oftentimes, the situations and people in our life that are causing the most stress and pain are there to remind us that we are not following our heart. This can come in the form of an angry boss at a job we hate or an abusive partner in a relationship that is not working.

If you are afraid of the changes that will happen in your life as a result of following your heart, that's natural. Just surrender to the changes, letting them happen. Don't resist them, don't tense up; just relax and allow them to happen. You are following your heart, which means you are finally having the experiences your soul desires. This also means you are getting back on the right path and living your life's purpose. The universe is ready to reward you.

There will be a transition stage as you move from where you are *not supposed* to be in life to where you *are supposed* to be. It's awkward, but you can't avoid this stage. Just like after surgery, there's a period of time when your body is healing and you may feel some discomfort. But surgery can save your life and so can following your heart. Anytime you experience any transitional discomfort, just relax and say these words to yourself: "This is my heart's desire, and I allow these changes to take place in my life."

The changes that took place in my life when my body was transforming itself were substantial to say the least. Allowing those changes to take place was the single greatest thing I have ever done. The rewards have been beyond my wildest expectations.

Update—I've since lost touch with Gina, but I heard from a mutual friend that she's lost weight and is doing fabulously as an artist and just had her first big art exhibit.

Mental Obesity: Beliefs That Get In The Way

What I call "mental obesity" is when your beliefs either cause you to gain weight or prevent you from losing weight. To a much larger extent than people would like to admit, our beliefs create and affect our reality. If beliefs are useful, they make everything flow smoothly. But dysfunctional beliefs only get in the way, and you may need to reexamine them, update them, or acquire new beliefs.

I once heard of a railway worker in Canada who worked on a train that had refrigerated cars. His greatest fear was that he would accidentally be locked in one of the cars one day and that he would freeze to death. Sure enough, one day he was inadvertently locked into one of these cars. He wrote a letter to his daughter about how he was always afraid of this happening, and he died in the car that night. The next day they found his body, and the coroner's report stated that he had indeed frozen to death. The only problem with what would have otherwise been an obvious diagnosis was that the refrigeration in the car *wasn't turned on that night.* He had frozen to death simply because he *believed* that he was going to freeze to death.

A well-known phenomenon in Australia is the aboriginal practice of "pointing the bone." A medicine man will point at his victim with a sharpened bone extracted from the body of a goanna (a species of giant monitor lizard) or a kangaroo.

Victims believe so strongly in the power of the bone that they quickly sicken and refuse to eat or drink. Unless a Ngangkari healer intervenes, they die, victims of their own beliefs. "Pointing the bone" works because it's common knowledge—an accepted belief—that the bone is fatal. It works and has done so for thousands of years. People die because they truly *believe* the bone will kill them. If beliefs can kill, then there is little question they have the power to activate and deactivate the FAT Programs too.

Beliefs can control our entire reality because they act like reality filters. If we believe something is possible or will happen, we open up a range of possibilities to allow particular realities to occur. On the other hand, if we think that something is difficult or impossible to accomplish, we shut ourselves off from the possibilities, thus almost ensuring that an event will not occur. The harder we think something is to achieve, the harder achieving it will become. As the saying goes, argue for your limitations and sure enough they're yours. However, the easier we think something is to achieve, the easier we make it for ourselves.

People kill and die for their beliefs, and yet, personally, I couldn't care less if my beliefs are "right" or "wrong." I only ever ask myself one question: "Does this belief serve me and those with whom I share my planet?" If so, then I keep it; if not, it's out. It's that simple.

When it comes to weight loss, you may have tried and failed so many times that you have come to believe that losing weight is either extremely difficult or downright impossible. I would urge you to allow yourself to release these negative beliefs; they will only get in your way. Believing that losing weight is difficult—for whatever reason—causes mental obesity.

Losing weight, in fact, is quite easy. Up until now, you've simply gone about it the wrong way. Whatever previous failure you've had has not been your fault; you've simply been using ineffective methods. Anyone using ineffective methods to achieve any goal will fail. That's what makes them ineffective. That's why diets have such a miserable success rate.

Every time you stick your hand in a fire, you'll get burned, and every time you try to lose weight by violating your body's natural logic, your body will fight you. Once you start using *effective* strategies for weight loss, you will lose weight easily and effortlessly.

Why let old, dysfunctional beliefs get in the way?

You *can* remove the beliefs that are causing mental obesity by re-educating your mind. You can turn beliefs on and off like a light switch to suit your needs. And we'll be talking about that soon enough. But the easier you believe it is for you to lose weight, the easier it becomes. You can use the power of beliefs to your advantage.

In a little while, I'll give you a set of highly effective tools to address mental starvation and mental obesity, but first, let's turn our attention to the most important nonphysical cause of obesity there is: emotional obesity.

NOTES

1. See S. Talbott, *The Cortisol Connection* (Alameda, CA: Hunter House Publishers, 2002).

2. See C. Ryff, "Study: Good Health Goes Beyond Diet and Exercise," University of Wisconsin–Madison Website (August 12, 2004): http://www.news.wisc.edu/10034.

4

Emotional Obesity

When you have emotional obesity, you've drawn the conclusion, either consciously or unconsciously, that being fat makes you feel safer. When this happens, you're sending the message to your body that being fatter is the best way to protect you from emotional stresses in your life.

Emotional Obesity Versus Emotional Eating

Emotional obesity is different from emotional eating. Emotional eating happens when you've formed an association between food and some positive emotional state, such as love, joy, happiness, security, or safety. It's the classic "comfort food" scenario when we use eating as emotional support, as fun and entertainment, or simply for the pleasure of it all.

Emotional eating is something everyone does to some degree, especially in cultures where people value the preparation and sharing of food. Emotional eating might, at first glance, explain why some people are fat, but I know a lot of emotional eaters who enjoy food, associate it with love and comfort, eat whatever they want, and aren't overweight. Simply put, their bodies don't want to be fat.

In general, eating for any reason other than nutrition is a form of emotional eating.

Emotional obesity, on the other hand, is the actual need to be fat, whether consciously or subconsciously, as an emotional survival strategy. You could, in theory, have no positive associations with food at all, and derive no pleasure from the act of eating, and still have emotional obesity—because it's not the food that's important, it's the fat.

Dealing with Emotional Obesity First

Whenever I talk with someone about their weight issues and I detect that they're showing signs of emotional obesity, I usually stop the conversation short and say to them, "Lets not talk about what you're eating or not eating right now, or how many times you've tried to diet and failed, or what you're cravings are or what type of exercise you're doing, or when you're 'good' or when you're 'bad.' I think that you have an emotional need to be fat, and as long as you have that need, no program is going to work for you. Let's first discover and understand why you have this need to be fat, and then see what we can do to eliminate that need."

Only after they have made some progress in addressing and eliminating the causes of their emotional obesity do I then say to them, "Okay, now I'm ready to discuss your eating habits; your cravings; your energy level; and what's hard or easy about your life in general, and about losing weight in particular. From there we can go about designing an approach that addresses and eliminates the reasons your body wants to be fat."

More times than not, I find that once people deal with the emotional obesity issue, their weight just falls off, and I don't hear from them again for several months.

Basically, it's futile to discuss any type of strategies for losing weight if you have mental and/or emotional reasons why you need to be fat—unless you *address these issues*.

Even the simplest and most effortless approach to weight loss will fail if you have emotional obesity. Someone could say to you, "All you need to do is lift your little finger once a day for thirty days straight in order to lose weight," but if you're in the grip of emotional obesity, you'll find some reason why it wasn't possible to complete the program. You'll "forget" or you "won't have time," or "other things will just get in the way." You'll sabotage your weight-loss effort because, at some level, the need to be fat serves a vitally important survival function in your life.

The Themes of Emotional Obesity

Any intrusion of your "boundaries" can cause emotional obesity because the fat can symbolically widen your boundaries. Fat can create distance between you and the person, thing, or situation that is infringing on your space. All forms of abuse, whether physical, mental, or emotional, are violations of boundaries.

Mental and Emotional Abuse

Emotionally abusive relationships—those with people who are controlling, interrogating, and dominating—are forms of violation of your mental and emotional "space."

Bill, a former associate of mine who knew me when I was fat, saw recent pictures of me and asked, "Is that the *real* you that was hiding behind a couple of hundred pounds of extra fat?" And I thought to myself, yes, that's the real me and that's exactly what I was doing: hiding behind a couple of hundred extra pounds of fat.

While I was working on Wall Street, I had a very close working relationship with someone who was extremely aggressive. Even though I loved and respected him, he also terrified me. This is probably my deepest, darkest secret that I'm about to share with you. It's hard for a grown man to admit that he's afraid of another person. It didn't matter that my fear was totally irrational and unfounded, but I admit that there was not a single moment when I was in this person's presence that I was not terrified.

He was very intelligent and he was a brilliant debater. He was constantly interrogating me and picking fights with me. He would be angry sometimes for days at a time, and I simply never felt safe in his presence, not for one single moment—ever! *This working relationship lasted for ten years.*

Around him, I always felt as if he was violating my mental space. Our working relationship was such that we were both very much dependent on each other for the success of our business. I needed him as much as he needed me. As a result, there was nowhere to run, nowhere to hide.

Because I could not escape, the only thing I could do was try to create some kind of distance between the two of us, and that is exactly what I did. The fat created distance between us; in essence, I was hiding inside my body. The fat acted like a buffer zone between us, and it very much made me feel safer.

The fat also made me feel safer because, the bigger I was, the less threatening he seemed to be. He was already taller and stronger than me, and this made me afraid of him physically. Sometimes when he was angry, he would start flailing his arms around and throwing things, and I was always afraid that the situation would get violent.

In his defense, he never got violent nor did he have a violent nature. But I was still always afraid that we would come to blows. Eventually, I was literally twice his size. Once I got big enough, I knew that he wouldn't attack me in a million years.

The way my body adapted was very similar to what happens in nature. Animals that can't run away from predators sometimes just get so big that no predator will touch them. Look at elephants or whales. They can't outrun predators, but they also don't have to worry about them because nothing is ever going to try to attack them. I couldn't run away from my attacker, so I became like a whale instead.

If you are in an abusive relationship of any kind, you need to get help from family, friends, loved ones, or professionals. The relationship has to either change or end. Sometimes, once you are able to express yourself to your abuser, he or she will become aware of the dynamic and change. In most cases, when it comes to emotional abuse, the abuser has no idea what is going on in your head.

Don't discount your feelings by sweeping them under the carpet, because it's these feelings that are making and keeping you fat. If you want to lose weight, the nature of the relationship must change and your feelings about the relationship must change as well. You simply must be able to feel safe around everyone in your life. This is your birthright, and if you don't have it right now, you must reclaim it.

Start by acknowledging your feelings. They are real, they are important, and they must be expressed. Talk to people that you do feel safe around until you understand your feelings well enough to be able to express them to your abuser in an effective manner. It's possible that both of you may need counseling or mediation with a third party to work out the issues.

Sometimes, just recognizing that your fear is causing you to be fat is all it takes to resolve emotional obesity. It may not make your relationship difficulties go away, but it will stop making you fat.

Physical and Sexual Abuse

In the case of physical abuse, when your physical boundaries are being violated, fat creates a boundary and a shield between you and the abuser in the same way that it does with emotional abuse. Fat literally puts the abuser farther away. Sometimes, in the case of sexual abuse, when you get fat *enough,* the abuser loses all interest in molesting someone who is hundreds of pounds overweight.

Many people have related to me sad stories of their childhood abuse and how, once they became so fat, the abuser moved on. In this case, the fat really did protect them. Unfortunately, it also left a nearly indelible imprint on their subconscious. I say "nearly" indelible because it does not have to be indelible; there are things that you can do to permanently remove the association between being fat and being protected.

If you have been abused in the past, your unresolved feelings might still be influencing you, causing you not to trust people and to have emotional obesity. Later in this chapter and at the end of this section, we'll talk about some ways of reeducating yourself so that you can once again feel safe and protected. You *can* liberate yourself from the shackles of emotional obesity.

Obviously, if you are currently being physically or sexually abused, you must get help immediately. It has to end and it has to end *now*! You must get as much help as you need in order to feel safe and protected from the abuse, including getting the law involved. Your legal rights are being violated, and you have every right to legal protection. You need to *be* safe and, as far as weight loss is concerned, you need to *feel* safe.

Hiding from the World

While fear makes some people fat, it makes others painfully thin. I once read an interview with a former anorexic in which she said that she wanted to become invisible to the world. She felt that, by being as small as possible, people would not notice her.

When I read this article, it occurred to me that gaining weight is a way of hiding from the world too. The same way that a turtle has a protective shell that it can hide in whenever something's attacking it, it's possible to make the association that our fat is a protective shell that can enable us to hide from threats in our lives.

This is a perfect example of how people can adopt opposite strategies for dealing with the same need—in this case, the need is to hide. One way of hiding is to become less visible; the other involves retreating *inside* your body—underneath your fat.

It's not the objective reality of the threat that matters; it's the way your body interprets the threat that determines its reaction.

One person's body can translate the need to hide into a need to be as thin a possible. Another person's body will interpret the need to hide as a need to be as fat as possible, causing them to become "morbidly" obese (I hate that term!). It's the exact same need with exactly opposite strategies for coping.

Big Is Boss

As children, we make the obvious connection that adults are in charge. Subconsciously, the association between "big" and "boss" still exists in us. Many people find that they're more comfortable in the role of an authority figure if they're bigger. We can also make the connection between being big physically and being *important*. An important person is a "big" man—the Big Chief, the Big Cheese, or the Big Dog. Policemen, for example, often feel safer being bigger because size and weight carry the illusion of authority.

Self-Punishment

We may want to be fat to punish ourselves because we don't feel that we are worthy of success, a beautiful body, love, or the respect of others or ourselves. If we are angry with ourselves or if we don't like ourselves, being fat is a method of punishment.

I read a story in the *New York Times* about a 400-pound man who trekked across the United States to lose weight. He hadn't always been fat; in fact, he had once been a fit marine. However, fourteen years before this walk, at the age of twenty-five, he had killed two people in a car accident.

The people who died had gotten off a bus at a bad intersection, and the man couldn't see them. In terrible remorse over the months and years that followed, he gained more and more weight. The extreme, chronic stress had activated his FAT Programs, and fat was his self-inflicted punishment. But perhaps his cross-country walk was a sign that he had punished himself enough, that he had "paid his dues," and that he was now ready to move on.

Rebellion

If your family is preoccupied with health and fitness, gaining weight may be a form of personal rebellion. You may be communicating to your family: "I am depriving you of the satisfaction you would derive from me being thin."

Rebellion is always about power and control. Everybody wants a healthy level of control over their own lives, so it's not surprising that some people will use obesity as a way of asserting themselves. If somebody else wants you to lose weight or is forcing you to lose weight, you may want to stay fat just so that you can reassert control over your life.

Dieting has always been an issue in my family. My father was heavy as a child and so was my brother (I was actually skinny as a kid). My father did not want my brother to suffer the pain that he experienced growing up, so he did everything in his power to try and help my brother lose weight. However well-meaning his intentions were, it only served to make my brother feel powerless over his own eating.

I remember when we were kids, my brother told me that every time he had some spare change, he would buy junk food with the deliberate aim of getting the most calories for his money.

Parents, children, husbands, and wives should be aware that nagging sends a couple of harmful messages:

- "You're not okay the way you are."
- "I know better than you what's good for you."

Nagging can lead to resentment and a desire to stay fat in order to make a point. One thing that I'm eternally grateful for is that, while I was gaining weight, my spouse never said a word about it, which I think is pretty incredible. I believe this made it much easier for me when I was finally ready to lose weight. And you can't force people to lose weight anyway; they lose weight when they're ready. This applies especially to children.

Testing Love: Pushing Our Loved Ones Away

If we think that someone loves us, not for ourselves but for what we have, it's logical to get rid of what we have to see if they still stick around through the "for richer or poorer" phases of our lives. If we think that someone only loves us for our looks, we may wish to test that love by seeing if they still love us no matter how we look. We may also want to push our partners away because we feel unlovable, or because they are being too demanding emotionally or in the bedroom.

If you're a new mother, you may feel like you just "need a little space," both from your children and your husband. I find this to be very common. You may love your family with all your heart, wanting only to give and give, but if you don't find a way to replenish yourself, you can run out of energy. You need some time and space just for you, and if you don't get it, your body will try to give you that space by creating a buffer between you and your life. It does this the only way it can: by creating a buffer of fat that protects you from the outside world.

Becoming Unlovable and "The Betrayal"

If you feel that losing weight will alienate you from your loved ones in any way, you'll want to stay fat. You might be in a marriage where you're losing weight, but your spouse isn't. This may bring up all sorts of tensions. Your spouse could get jealous that you've become more attractive, or he or she might feel threatened because "Being fat is good enough for me. Why isn't it good enough for you?"

It's possible that your spouse prefers your being fat. If you feel that your spouse is attracted to you because you're heavy, you have a powerful disincentive to losing weight. It could also be, for example, that everybody in your family is fat and that, if you became thin, you wouldn't be "family" anymore. You would then be "betraying" your family.

You need to be aware that, as you lose weight, your relationships with people may change. If you're afraid of those changes, you may stay heavy simply not to "rock the boat." But if not "rocking the boat" is an important point for you, either consciously or subconsciously, you'll be fighting this fear unless you eliminate it. Yes, you can eliminate these sorts of fears, and I'll cover how to do that shortly.

Grief

If someone we love leaves us, either through separation or death, we often feel a lack of control over the situation. In an effort to hold on to that person, we may want to gain weight.

Cheryl had a daughter, Michelle, who died of a brain tumor when she was eight. This was a very emotionally demanding and devastating experience for Cheryl. After Michelle's death, Cheryl gained 63 pounds—Michelle's *exact* weight at the time of her death. Cheryl was trying, in vain, to keep Michelle physically with her always.

But Cheryl now understands the real issue with her weight and, rather than dieting (something she has been doing for over thirty years), she is dealing with the real issues more directly. As a matter of fact, she wrote a book about her experience. It's a poignant story, full of courage and triumph in the face of adversity, and if you're dealing with deep issues, such as this one, you might find writing about it helps too.

Using Fat as an Excuse

A young man who called me believed that no one would hire him because he was "morbidly" obese. He felt that, in order for him to be employable, he had to first lose weight. I realized that as long as he had this idea, he would not lose weight. He was using his weight as an excuse not to work. He had certain issues about work and about being employable, and he was using his weight as a convenient excuse to avoid these issues.

We also may use weight to avoid facing the issues of relationships. If someone claims that they need to lose weight before starting to date or embarking on a relationship, they may unconsciously be using their weight to avoid facing other relationship issues. It's easier to blame the fat than to confront the issues. As long as we are using our weight to avoid other uncomfortable aspects of our lives, we'll resist losing the weight because it's become the scapegoat that's distracting others and ourselves from what's really going on.

Issues from Past Lives

Some people believe that we have lived before and others don't. It doesn't matter to me what you believe, but if you do believe in past lives, you might entertain the idea that your weight issues could be related to a previous life. Dr. Brian Weiss, in one of his fascinating books about past life regression,[1] told a story about a woman who could not lose weight. It was discovered during a past life regression that she had been abused and had made the connection that she was less likely to be abused again if she was overweight. Once she came to this understanding, she was able to release her weight issues.

Another past life story I've heard is about a man who previously lived in a culture where being fat was synonymous with being rich and powerful. As a result, his soul in this life expressed a desire to be fat because he made the association that being fat is desirable. I also once heard about a lady who found that, in her past lives, she relied on her body to help her get what she wanted too many times. In this life, she chose to be fat so that she would not rely on her body as a tool of persuasion. When she was able to make this realization, her weight issues went away.

I find that people with past life issues surrounding their weight are often very curious about their former lives. It's as if something just resonates inside them when they hear about the possibility that their weight issues could be related to events in their distant pasts.

Trauma

Any trauma, particularly serious trauma, may make you feel that the world is unsafe and therefore trigger emotional obesity. I had a friend who was in a serious motorcycle accident, and after he got out of hospital, all he wanted to do for the next six months was stay in his room and eat. Divorce, job loss, and even witnessing someone else's trauma may cause emotional obesity.

Overcoming Emotional Obesity Due to Trauma and Abuse

If you can trace the onset of your weight gain to a specific incident in your life, such as being abused as a child; being in a car accident; undergoing a divorce; or experiencing the separation of your parents, a loved one dying or leaving you, a past life, or any other trauma, I strongly recommend that you enlist the services of a qualified therapist. There are many excellent healing modalities around. Find one that appeals to you, and spend some time working though the issues and releasing the pain. This will allow you to move forward and relcase emotional obesity. Some of the therapies I've found to be effective are Core Energetics, Soul Retrieval, and regression analysis. Please see my website gabrielmethod.com for a list of recommended counselors in your area.

But I really have to make this point very strongly: if you're not addressing these issues, you're not following the Gabriel Method. No one can say for sure how long it will take before the issues are resolved; that process is deeply personal. The issues might be resolved at this very moment, simply by reading this chapter or by listening to my CD once, or it might take months of intensive counseling. There's simply no way to predict what it will take, but starting the process is the key.

At least there's a really easy way to know something for sure right now. Ask yourself a simple question: "Do I feel safe being thin?" If the answer is no, then there's still a problem. Can you imagine yourself being thin? If not, you are not quite there yet, but don't worry. I will help you work on getting there in the coming chapters. Also, if someone comments on how great you look and how thin you're getting, does that make you feel happy or threatened? If it makes you feel uncomfortable in the slightest, that is a sign.

In the coming chapters, I talk about some very effective ways of addressing and eliminating the causes of emotional obesity, but only you will know for sure if it's working for you and the extent to which you need to keep going in this area.

You can take care of emotional obesity easily enough, but you must take care of it. You simply cannot ignore it. If you have it, no diet, program, or approach will be effective. Rather than ignore the problem, address it and watch the weight literally melt off your body.

You will know when your emotional obesity is gone because you will feel safer, more centered, less fearful, calmer, happier, more open, more positive, and more in control of you life. These positive emotional states may happen gradually or all at once as you address and resolve your emotional obesity issues.

You will no longer need to be fat in order to feel safe. Your body will turn off the FAT Programs, and it will actually start helping you lose weight.

So now that we've talked about the many mental and emotional stresses that can activate the FAT Programs, let's turn our attention toward what we can do to eliminate them.

NOTES

1. See B. Weiss, *Many Lives, Many Masters* (New York: Simon & Schuster/Fireside Press, 1988).

5

Eliminating the Nonphysical Causes of Obesity Using SMART Mode™

The stress signals that can trick your body into activating FAT Programs all originate from negative emotions, such as fear, sadness, longing, anger, and resentment. If you have no fear, you have no stress. Negative emotions communicate to your body that there is some form of threat out there—that in some way you are not safe.

But you can eliminate negative emotions by going to the source of these feelings. After all, we have to create our emotions; they don't just come out of nowhere. Beliefs generate emotions. For example, one simple dysfunctional belief, such as "everyone hates me," can generate negative emotions all day long. On the other hand, a more positive belief, such as "I'm safe," can make us happy and content for an entire lifetime. Change your beliefs, and you instantly and permanently transform your emotional state.

Let's look at an example as it applies to weight loss. Imagine that you have arbitrarily decided at some conscious or subconscious level that being fat is in some way making you safer. As you know, holding this belief is a problem that is going to undermine your efforts no matter how hard you struggle and force yourself to lose weight.

Until you let it go, this belief will always be there. If you were simply able to change your thinking so that instead you believed that the thinner you are, the safer you are, your weight problems would be solved.

One simple thought, one simple change, and weight loss becomes effortless.

Now, you don't have to be *totally* fearless in order to lose weight; it's enough to simply focus on those thoughts that are causing the problems. This is something that is really very easy to do, and it can happen instantly. But you have to understand one thing: you can't easily make changes to your thinking in your normal waking state, or what's known as the "beta" state of consciousness. Changing "wrong" thinking is not going to happen by making a conscious effort or by an act of will. You *have* to enter a state of awareness in which you can actually make the appropriate changes and have them stay with you for life.

I call this particular state of awareness "Super Mental Awareness Re-education Training Mode," or SMART Mode.

When you are in SMART Mode, you become a super-learning machine. You can make quick and permanent changes to your thinking. SMART Mode allows your brain to reach very relaxing and pleasant states of awareness, which experts call "alpha" and "theta" states. These are perfectly normal, natural states you pass through every night as you are going to sleep. The only difference is that SMART Mode happens when you enter this state consciously.

That's why I made the evening visualization CD.[1] The first thing the CD does is relax you and put you in SMART Mode. Once you're in SMART Mode, the CD makes certain extremely beneficial suggestions targeted toward eliminating the nonphysical causes of obesity.

What happens then is, while you sleep, your subconscious integrates these suggestions into your thinking until they become an automatic part of your everyday life. An added bonus is that the CD will also help you get a great night's sleep.

Transform your body while you sleep. It doesn't get any better than that! You get to sleep deeply and gain all the rest you need, while your subconscious is solving your problems for you—forever. This is the most effective, effortless way of solving your weight-loss problems.

SMART Mode is similar to the state of awareness you are in when meditating. It's the state that artists achieve when they are in the state of flow and that state that brilliant inventors achieve when they're touched by inspiration. Albert Einstein spent much of his time in SMART Mode.

You also enter this state when you are painting, fishing, in "the zone" during a sporting event, watching an extremely captivating performance, or at any time when you are either highly focused or very relaxed. Children spend a great deal of their time in SMART Mode; that's why they're so impressionable and why they can learn things so quickly. And if you don't think that your kids are smart, ask yourself why they have the ability to learn a second language without a trace of an accent.

If you don't want to listen to the CD, you can still get into SMART Mode and make whatever changes you want. Here's a really quick, easy way you can get into SMART Mode on your own:

Spinning the Spine for Getting Into SMART Mode

"Spinning the Spine" is one of the most effective techniques I've found for getting into SMART Mode. Its beauty lies in its simplicity.

- Go into a room where you'll not be disturbed for about ten minutes.
- Sit with your spine straight and your eyes closed, and imagine a tiny beam of light circling around the first vertebra at the base of your spine. Each time the beam of light circles around your first vertebra, count until the tiny beam of light has circled ten times.
- Imagine moving the tiny beam of light to the second vertebra and circling ten times. Count from eleven to twenty as it circles this vertebra.

- Then imagine that the beam of light moves up to the third vertebra and circles around this vertebra ten times. Count from twenty-one to thirty as it circles the third vertebra.
- There are twenty-four vertebra in the spine. So by circling around each vertebra ten times and counting from zero to two hundred forty, you will have traveled up your entire spine. Two hundred forty seconds is four minutes, so this technique should take approximately four to five minutes.

Don't worry about the exact location of each vertebra. Just know that if you are counting from 150 to 160, for example, your attention should be where you would imagine your sixteenth vertebra to be. I would imagine that to be in the middle part of my spine. When you get to two hundred, your attention should be around the base of the neck.

You'll notice that as you move up your spine, your mind starts to become calmer and more focused.

Music for Getting into SMART Mode

There are many companies that make music recordings specially geared toward putting you into a more focused, creative state of being. All you have to do is listen to the music and your brain will automatically go into SMART Mode. Please check my website gabrielmethod.com for a list of suggested music recordings from different companies that provide this service.

Using Power Words in SMART Mode

When you're in SMART Mode, saying simple words and phrases can be very effective in totally transforming the way you think and feel. I call these words and phrases "power words" because, when you use them in SMART Mode, they have the power to quickly become part of your everyday thinking.

It's really simple. While in SMART Mode, simply imagine any word or phrase that you would like to adapt as a way of thinking. Then picture the word or phrase actually winding up your spine. As it winds up your spine, imagine that it is charging every cell of your body with its intention.

Here are some examples of power words that have worked for me:

For Less Stress

- Relax
- Life is easy
- Life is flow
- All is good
- Life is working
- Everything's good

For Changing the Feeling of Lack and Limitation

- Infinite abundance
- Abundance flows to me
- I am always taken care of

For Emotional Obesity

- Safe
- I am safe
- Thin is safe
- Life is safe
- I feel safe

For Mental Obesity

- Effortless weight loss
- Weight loss is easy
- My body wants to be thin
- Excess weight melts off my body
- I am naturally thin
- I am effortlessly thin

By saying power words in SMART Mode, you're reprogramming the way you think so you have less stress, and fewer fears and dysfunctional thoughts that can trick your body into activating the FAT Programs.

Eventually, powerful, positive emotions will become an automatic part of your daily life so that all day, without your having to think about it, you will be eliminating the stress signals that were sabotaging your body into thinking that it needed to be fat. Your body will then turn off the FAT Programs, and weight loss will become automatic.

The next chapter talks about some highly effective visualizations you can practice while you are in SMART Mode. These visualizations will enable you to eliminate the causes of mental and emotional obesity, and create the body of your dreams.

NOTES

1. Please go to http://www.gabrielmethod.com/cd for instructions on how to download *The Gabriel Method Evening Visualization* CD for free.

6

Using Positive Emotions to Turn Off the FAT Programs

If you can develop the habit of automatically thinking positively, you'll be able to cut out 90 percent of the stress signals that trick your body into thinking that you're not safe and that you need to be fat in order to be protected. Thoughts are habits; the more we think a certain way, the more we reinforce those thinking habits.

You may be in the habit of thinking negatively, and being angry and fearful without even being aware of it. As a result, while you are driving to work, while you are making dinner, while you are getting dressed—in fact all day long—you are sending the following stress signal to your body: "I am not safe! Do something! I am not safe! Do something! I am not safe! Do something!"

Your body doesn't know exactly what do to, but for some of us, it turns on the FAT Programs. If that happens, you've got a problem.

However, thinking positively is also a habit; the more you do it, the more ingrained it becomes. By being in the habit of positive thinking, you'll be doing away with the stress signals that are tricking your brain into turning on the FAT Programs.

The Power of Your Positive Emotions

Creating the habit of positive thinking is one-stop shopping for automatically eliminating nearly all forms of mental and emotional obesity that confuse your body into thinking you need to be fat. Consider this:

- When you're a habitually-positive thinker, the stress of the daily grind doesn't affect you as much—so you generate fewer *mental starvation* signals.
- You're nourishing yourself with positive emotions and your life is more fun—so you generate fewer *emotional starvation* signals.
- You feel more connected to the world, and your life has more purpose and meaning—so you generate fewer *spiritual starvation* signals.
- You feel safer, you have less fear, and life becomes less threatening. You open up to the world and feel more in control. You also feel less angry and less inclined to use fat as a shield or as a weapon—you no longer suffer from *emotional obesity*.
- You're less likely to give power to negative beliefs that hold you back—so you don't have *mental obesity*.

Below are a few very useful techniques for creating the habit of thinking positively. The more you practice them, the more automatic positive thinking will become. Not only will you enable your body to lose weight, you'll also be transforming your mind into a positive energy generator. This energy will then influence and power every other aspect of your life as well.

Techniques for Lightening Your Load

Radiating Love

Love is the ultimate positive emotion to lighten your energy. It makes your life smoother, easier, more satisfying, more meaningful, and more enjoyable.

Technique: Sit alone quietly and use this imagery: imagine the feeling of a gentle, loving kiss of sunlight around your heart.[1] Feel this loving kiss of light bathe your heart and then imagine that it radiates out in every direction. Feel this light illuminate, nourish, and charge every cell of your body with love. After a few minutes, imagine that the light shines like a spotlight radiating from the center of your chest, illuminating and energizing everything it touches.

Fill the room you're in and then the trees, plants, and flowers outside with this love. Let the light continue to expand in all directions until it encompasses the whole Earth, solar system, galaxy, universe, and beyond.

In your everyday life, whenever you think of it, imagine this spotlight of love emanating from your heart. I've noticed that the second I start to project this loving vibration out into the world, the situation that I'm in instantly becomes easier and more pleasant. This works whether I'm in a stressful or difficult situation, or whether I'm confronting a difficult or negative person.

Radiate Forgiveness

One of the highest states of being is that of universal forgiveness. Life is challenging for everyone. We are all trying to satisfy our needs in one way or another, and we are all doing the best we can with the understanding that we have. Everyone has selfish needs and noble needs. Sometimes one person's understanding of how they can best satisfy their needs infringes on another person's needs, wants, desires, or rights. This is inevitable. We've all been hurt and we've all hurt others. Some hurts are inexcusable; however, blaming others and failing to forgive them serves no one, least of all you.

Forgiveness is an act of letting go, an act of release. We release the pain, the hurt, and the wrong. When we are able to release all of this emotional baggage, we are then able to release our physical baggage in the form of excess weight.

Judging yourself is just as bad as judging someone else. Our thoughts are a powerful force, and what you pay attention to you empower. Judging yourself only serves to strengthen your shortcomings.

Forgiveness is a magnanimous act. It makes you feel good about yourself, which makes you feel more deserving of good. When you feel more deserving, you are more able to give yourself the gift of the body you desire.

Technique: Sit alone quietly and say the word FORGIVENESS. Say it slowly several times. Imagine every cell of your body is saying the word in unison. After a while, certain people will come to mind that you need to forgive. As people arise in your awareness, say that you forgive them. Imagine that every cell of your body forgives them. Don't forget to include yourself.

Radiate Appreciation

It's impossible to have negative thoughts while feeling appreciation. Appreciation dissolves negativity. Where there is appreciation, there can never be sadness, anger, resentment, and those other poisonous emotions that trigger the FAT Programs.

There's an opportunity to feel appreciation in every situation. Even if you're in a traffic jam, that fundamental symbol of the daily grind, you can appreciate it. It may have made you ten minutes late, but you can be grateful that it didn't make you an hour late. You can be grateful that you weren't part of the accident that caused the traffic jam in the first place, or that your car didn't stall on the freeway.

There is an infinite number of things that we can all appreciate once we start to think about it. You can choose to find gratitude in every moment and to develop this habit of appreciation in every circumstance.

I have found that whenever I am in a challenging situation in my life, if I utter the statement "I am grateful for the grace of this moment," the situation is almost magically transformed. For me this has become a habit, and it has made my life infinitely easier and less stressful.

Technique: In the same way as the previous technique, sit alone quietly and say the word APPRECIATION. Say it slowly several times. Feel every cell of your body joining in the chorus. After a while, things and people will come to mind for you to appreciate. As each thing or person comes to mind, feel your appreciation for each one.

Your body might come to mind. Say: "I APPRECIATE MY BODY." Perhaps some aspect of your relationships or your career or your life will come to mind. Appreciate these things too.

You can also practice this technique by saying: "I AM GRATEFUL."

Accept the Negative

I once read in Ken Wilber's book *No Boundary* that, if you want to get rid of any offensive aspect of yourself, and all those shadowy, negative thoughts and feelings that creep up, the best way to do it is to accept them and integrate them into your consciousness. Wilber says these are aspects of yourself that you have rejected and alienated from what you think of as the real you. They are like naughty children that intentionally cause problems because they want some attention, even if it's negative attention.

These thoughts can cause all kinds of negative feelings. We can't believe nice people could think such things, so we then judge ourselves as horrible people for having such miserable thoughts. But the more we fight and resist our negative thoughts, the more they pop up. This is because we are rewarding them with negative attention. If we reward children with negative attention whenever they do something wrong, they'll continue to behave badly because negative attention is better than no attention at all. It's the same with our thoughts.

But according to Wilber, the answer is to acknowledge these thoughts as a part of ourselves and to integrate them instead of alienating them. By doing so, the thoughts are satisfied, they feel loved, and they stop behaving like naughty children.

Technique: Anytime that you have a negative thought, do not dwell on it. Simply say: "I acknowledge you and I accept you," then feel the thought instantly dissolve. Concentrate on the relief and relaxation that your body feels as it releases tension from each and every cell.

Accept Your Body Exactly as It Is

It's important to come to a point where you feel you're comfortable with your body exactly as it is right now. One of the things that helped me tremendously in the beginning was coming to a place mentally where I decided that I could live the rest of my life exactly as I was (and this was when I weighed over 400 pounds!), but I just didn't want to gain any more weight. Once I came to this place in my thinking, I started losing weight.

As contrary as this may sound, rather than being dissatisfied and impatient with your weight, try being comfortable with yourself exactly as you are right now.

This is just another example of how accepting your negative aspects causes them to disappear. It's remarkable how effective this technique really is.

If you feel you're not all right exactly as you are and that you had better lose weight quickly, whether it's for a wedding or the swimsuit season or because you simply cannot stand yourself, you're effectively starving for self-esteem and self-acceptance. In essence, you're already on a diet, and as we know, *diets almost always fail.*

Throw Your Scales Away

Don't look at your scales for the first six months of your transformation!

This goes hand in hand with being okay exactly as you are right now. It's been my experience that the weight comes off in quantum leaps periodically. This means that you may be in plateaus for certain periods of time. If you weigh yourself every day, you can easily get discouraged during a plateau. But plateaus are important consolidation periods. Even though it may not be showing, a lot of things could be going on biochemically inside you that are getting you ready for the next big breakthrough.

Weighing yourself every day keeps the focus on how quickly you are losing weight. Take the focus off how quickly you're losing weight and focus instead on how effectively you are transforming your body permanently.

The Abundance Visualization

I love this visualization because it works on so many levels. Being worried about finances can activate the FAT Programs, as you now know. So, getting richer kills two birds with one stone: you solve your financial problems and you allow your body to let go of excess weight. I use visualization for everything in my life, and when it comes to creating more abundance, this visualization really hits the mark.

Technique: Imagine you are in an infinite ocean stretching as far as you can see in all directions. Even though you are in this ocean, you can still breathe just fine. Now imagine that this ocean is really an ocean of abundance, and that one drop of this water is equal to more money than Bill Gates can make in an entire lifetime—just one drop! You are completely submerged in it, and it goes as far as you can possibly imagine in all directions. Now, simply imagine that the pores of your skin are opening up, and that the water rushes into your body and then flows into your life. Imagine it flowing through you and creating any type of abundance you want—houses, cars, mansions, or just a general feeling of security. Affirm to yourself that you are always in this ocean, and anytime you need ANYTHING whatsoever, all you have to do is open your pores and allow it to flow to you.

What I like about this visualization is that it works on so many levels. When you do this visualization in SMART Mode, you're tapping into the enormous power of your mind to attract wealth, security, and abundance. You are communicating to your body that there is no need to store anything because there is no lack, so you begin to lose weight. And you are totally reprogramming the dysfunctional belief that you have to struggle to get wealth and abundance, allowing them to simply flow to you.

You cannot possibly imagine how effective this visualization is for making you feel less stress, for losing weight, and for actually increasing the flow of abundance into your life. I use it for any aspect of my life in which I feel lack. For example, when I want more love, I just imagine that the infinite ocean is actually an ocean of love, and then I open my pores and imagine love flowing in from all directions. I do this quite frequently, and I am always amazed at how much more loving the people in my life are to me afterwards.

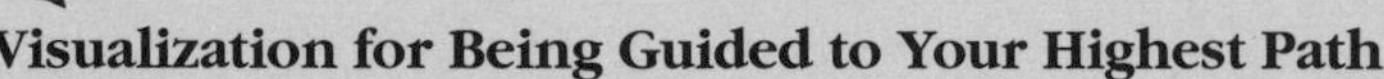

Visualization for Being Guided to Your Highest Path

Imagine you are on a raft that is flowing downstream. Just up ahead is the you of your dreams: a perfect body living the perfect life that you would like to be living. Then just relax and let go as you are naturally guided downstream toward your ideal life. As you get to your destination, step out of the raft and literally *step into* that body and that life. You are now living exactly the way you would like to live—according to your heart's desires—and you are doing it in your ideal body. You did all this simply by relaxing, letting go, and allowing yourself to be guided to your highest path.

Finding Your Passion

Many people have lost touch with joy and passion to such an extent that they are not even sure what it means to follow their heart. I know that's the way I once was. I was so exhausted that all I wanted to do was sleep, let alone live passionately. But what does following your heart mean to you? What makes you passionate? What do you live for? If you've forgotten, here's a great way to remember.

Technique: Imagine that you are waking up in a beautiful castle bedroom with a balcony overlooking the ocean. Imagine a large room with a canopied bed and white drapes gently blowing in a warm breeze.

For just this day, you are not a parent or someone's partner. You are infinitely wealthy, and you have no need to work. Everyone in your life is safe and taken care of. All deadlines are completed, and you have absolutely no responsibilities whatsoever. You have boundless energy, and you are in your most ideal shape. Everything is perfect.

A servant comes into the room with your breakfast and asks you what you would like to do today. Feel your answer. What *would* you like to do today? The answer is your passion; the answer is what your heart is calling you to do. Really connect to that and imagine yourself having that perfect day, enjoying every minute of it. Then, in your real life, during the day, try to incorporate some aspect of your vision into your life, even if it's just a symbolic gesture. Affirm that you will always follow your heart, and then surrender to that desire.

NOTES

1. See X. Waterkeyn, *Women In Crime* (Sydney: New Holland Publishers, 2005).

7

Creating the Body of Your Dreams

One of the fundamental problems everyone faces when trying to lose weight is that we don't know how to communicate with our own minds. Our conscious mind (what we generally think of as our mind) simply doesn't know how to communicate with our *unconscious* mind. The unconscious mind is the part of our mind that controls our animal brain.

The primary purpose of the animal brain is to keep us alive, safe, and healthy, and if we live long enough, it inspires us to procreate. It also controls our hunger and our body weight. The animal brain is very powerful and its role is crucial, yet there is one small problem: it doesn't understand the stresses of modern day living.

The animal brain understands life in terms of physical survival and simple dualities like safe/unsafe, run/fight, sleep/wake, eat more/eat less, get fatter/get thinner, and so on. In contrast, our conscious mind thinks in terms of ideas and concepts like "I'd like to lose 20 pounds so I can fit into my favorite dress and look good at my best friend's wedding next spring."

Trying to explain to the animal brain that you would like to look good for a wedding is a bit like trying to explain to a three year old that it's a good time to buy bank stocks while interest rates are going down. There are just too many concepts that are inconceivable to a young child.

In the same way, the animal brain doesn't know what a wedding is, or a dress, or looking good, or a best friend, or even next spring. It understands safe and unsafe, and all the myriad of chemical components that go into that equation.

Therefore, the basic challenge for all of us—a challenge that most of us are not even aware exists—is to simply learn how to communicate with our own brains. It's like being the owner of a beautiful estate when the estate manager only speaks ancient Greek and there are no translators.

That's why there are so many misunderstandings and why we often feel as if we are at war with our own bodies. You may *want* to be thin with all your heart at a *conscious* level, but your animal brain is holding all the cards. If it doesn't want you to be thin, because it doesn't understand that that's what *you* want or because it's under the mistaken impression that you need to be fat in order to be safe, then you're out of luck—plain and simple.

But what if you could learn to speak to your animal brain? What if you could find a way to communicate with it and explain to it that you don't want to be fat or need to be fat—that you actually want and need to be thin? If you make your animal brain understand that, it would quickly turn off the FAT Programs. After all, it's in *complete* control of your body, but it's also your willing servant. All you need to do is talk to it in a language it can understand, and all your problems are solved.

Fortunately, there is a way to do this.

Pictures—The Universal Language

Just as you can use pictures to communicate with someone who doesn't speak your language, you can use pictures—in the form of visualization—to communicate with your brain. Imagine you're in a foreign country, where you don't speak the language, and you need to do something basic, such as going to the toilet. You try asking someone where it is, but they don't understand you. You do some miming that you think makes it clear, but all you get is stares because they think that you're some kind of oddball. So what do you do? The obvious thing is to get a piece of paper and a pen, and draw a picture of a toilet.

The moment you show the picture to a friendly local, you've made your point. It doesn't matter if they only speak Swahili. If they've seen a toilet, they know exactly what you want and can point you in the right direction. Symbols and pictures are the universal language that everyone understands.

It's no different communicating to your own body. If you create a visual image of a thinner version of you, your brain will understand and work to make it happen.

Problem solved.

This is why visualization works so well. When you create a visual image of exactly how you want to look, you're basically programming yourself to look that way. You're talking to your unconscious mind and your animal brain, saying:

- I want to be thin.
- I need to be thin.
- You are getting the messages wrong.
- Turn off the FAT Programs, please.

More About SMART Mode

The key to successful and effective visualization is to perform visualization when you're in SMART Mode (see chapter 5).

When we are in SMART Mode, our internal chatter quiets down. Our ability to focus and create a visual image is much stronger, so the message that we are sending to our unconscious mind is much clearer. It's like looking at your reflection in a quiet pool of water. When the pool has no ripples, you can easily see your reflection as clearly as when you are looking into a mirror. But if there are waves in the water, your reflection becomes completely distorted. The unconscious mind is the same; when it is quiet, it becomes like a pool with no ripples. In this still state, it can understand the image you're creating and comprehend that it is what you want.

When the mind is racing, there are too many thought waves distorting the image; therefore, practicing visualization while you are in SMART Mode is the key to success. SMART Mode is the missing link in weight loss that has the power to transform your body into a body that *wants* to be thin.

Deepak Chopra has another explanation of why practicing visualization in SMART Mode is so effective. In his classic masterpiece *The Seven Spiritual Laws of Success*, he talks about both the "Law of Pure Potentiality" and the "Law of Intention and Desire." According to Dr. Chopra, we can manifest anything we want in our lives by taking intention or desire into the "field of pure potentiality."

The visual image of how you would like to look is the intention, and when you're in SMART Mode, you enter what Dr. Chopra calls the "field of pure potentiality." So according to this theory, by visualizing your ideal body in SMART Mode, you are manifesting that body—you are creating the *body of your dreams*.

I am living proof that this is true. The body that I now have is exactly the body that I visualized while I was losing weight. I don't believe this is a coincidence. It wasn't that I just lost weight; I now look *exactly* the way I pictured myself looking. When I weighed over 400 pounds, anyone seeing the picture of how I imagined myself looking would have laughed and said I was "dreaming"—*which of course I was*.

I was visualizing my ideal body in the powerful waking/dream state of SMART Mode.

As crazy as that image might have seemed to others, I clung to it and I *believed* in it, and now the dream has become a reality—just as it can become a reality for you too.

Another bonus of visualization is that, when you do it frequently, you'll actually start to *believe* you're going to look the way you're visualizing your body to be. We've talked about the tremendous power of beliefs in chapter 3, in the discussion of mental obesity. Specifically, we know that beliefs have the power to kill us or cure us, and we know that beliefs control nearly every aspect of our life experience. When you start to believe that you will look a certain way, you are tapping into the power of beliefs to make it happen. Even if, in the beginning, you may be visualizing without belief, eventually the belief will come, as will all the power you need to achieve it.

The beauty of the practice is that, once you are already in SMART Mode, it really only takes a minute to create the image.

Use the visualization techniques below so that the next time you're picturing your ideal body and someone comes along to say, "Yeah, right, in your dreams," you can reply: "Yes, in *my* dreams and coming soon to real life."

Making Visualization a Habit

It's important to make visualization a habit. When you do so, you'll be well on the way to transforming your body from the inside out.

Visualization becomes progressively easier over time. What may take you several minutes the first day may take only an effortless second or two by the end of the month. Once that happens, you have just acquired what is, in my opinion, possibly the most useful weight-loss asset you can have—the automatic, effortless habit of programming yourself to be thin.

Basic Visualization

You can practice this visualization any time, and I certainly encourage you to do so whenever you think about it. However, it is most effective when you are in SMART Mode, right before you go to sleep, or just as you are waking up.

Simply visualize yourself looking exactly the way you would like to look. That is all you really need to do. However, if you want to make it even more powerful, imagine that you are at a pleasant, scenic location.

For example, I used to visualize myself standing on top of a mountain, or walking or running on the beach. See yourself in your ideal shape, and imagine your body in the scene in as much detail as possible. Smell the air, feel the sun, hear the wind, taste and smell the salt of the ocean. See the scene as colorfully as possible—the blue and green hues of the ocean, the rich blue and bright white of the sky, the green fields or white snow-capped mountains ... whatever inspires you.

Be in the scene with *all* of your senses. Feel the way your body would feel if you were in perfect shape. See your skin having a healthy, vibrant glow. Imagine putting on suntan lotion and feeling the cool cream on your warm, toned, tight skin. See and feel the smooth coordination of your defined muscles as you put the lotion on your body. Notice how your toned, flat stomach glistens from the suntan lotion. Make the scene visceral and sensual. You are a beautiful, physical Amazon or Aphrodite, Adonis or Apollo. Your movements take on a sinewy, feline grace as you walk or run. While you're in the scene, say to yourself, "THIS IS ME," or you can say something like "I love my body" or maybe "I love being alive." Whatever you are saying, really *feel* it to be true.

Any type of visualization, whether you are in a scenic setting or not, will yield results, but the more you can use your imagination and your senses to bring you into the scene, the better it will work. However, if picturing an elaborate setting is too much effort, don't worry about it. Just imagine yourself being thin in any way that you can. Visualization will still work.

Other Visualizations That You Can Do

- **The Whirlpool**—Picture a whirlpool in your navel that it is sucking all the fat into it from all areas of your body. Imagine that all the fat on your body has been sucked into this whirlpool, never to be seen again.
- **The Fat Wash**—Imagine that a hose is spraying your body, and as it sprays your body, all the fat is washing off, just like dirt gets washed off a car. Visualize all the excess fat washing off and going into an imaginary drain in the floor, never to be seen again. This is also a great visualization to do while you are in the shower.

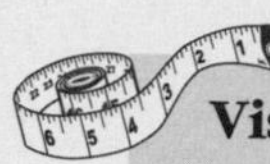

Visualizing While in Your Normal Waking State

You can visualize your body being in perfect shape throughout the day, whenever the idea occurs to you.

As you are watering the plants, for example, you can imagine that your body is in perfect shape. You can see that the muscles in your arms are perfectly defined and that your stomach is flat and lean.

When you're walking to work or as you're sitting in front of your computer, you can imagine that your body is in perfect shape.

8

Easy Applications of the Principles in Part II

Incorporating these SMART Mode concepts and actions into your life is very simple, though it may seem like an overwhelming amount of information. The key to this shift is using visualization.

All you need to do is develop the habit of practicing visualization at night, for a few minutes, just as you are about to go to sleep, and then listen to my CD just after that. The CD addresses *all* the issues discussed in this section—mental and emotional starvation, emotional obesity, mental obesity, and visualization.

If you don't want to listen to the CD, have a ten-minute SMART Mode visualization session sometime during the day, preferably first thing in the morning, right when you wake up. If you are *really* motivated, it's better to do both.

If you decide to do both, I suggest that you start by listening to the CD at night for a month and phase-in the SMART Mode visualization session in the second month.

Month One: The Basics of Visualization

Practice the following routine every morning and every evening for thirty consecutive days.

Find a picture of someone that looks exactly the way you would like to look. It could be you at an earlier time or it could be someone else, but the important thing is to find an image that closely resembles the body you'd like to create. Don't worry about any preconceptions you might have about whether or not it's "realistic" for you to look that way. Just assume anything is possible, and find the right image.

On the bottom of the picture, write the following statement (or something similar):

I use the power of my mind to create the body I desire.

Keep this picture in a handy place by your bed. Then before you go to sleep at night, do the following:

- Look at the picture for about thirty seconds.
- While staring at the picture, say the statement that you wrote on the bottom of the picture.
- Now close your eyes and imagine that you look exactly like the picture you were just staring at. You can to it for a few seconds or a few minutes, it's up to you.
- Expand that thought and imagine that you feel the way the image looks—whether it's running freely and lightly, dancing with joy, or even feeling your body as you try on smaller-size clothes. Let that feeling permeate your entire being.
- Play the CD and allow yourself to drift off to sleep while still listening to it.
- *The following morning*, while you're still lying in bed and before you get up, reach over to the picture, look at it for a few seconds, close your eyes, and visualize your ideal body once more.
- Spend a moment visualizing your coming day. Imagine it going exactly the way that you would like it to go, from start to finish.

Experts say that it takes twenty-one days to form a habit, so by doing this every day for a month, you will have formed a habit for life.

Month Two: The Daily Session

Once you have spent a month creating the habit of practicing visualization morning and evening, you can now focus on creating the habit of a daily SMART Mode session. This daily session is not absolutely necessary, but it is useful if you have the time and the inclination. The session should be around ten minutes long. Of course, the longer the better, and you may find that you really enjoy being in the state of SMART Mode. Many studies have shown that it reduces stress[1] and cortisol levels.[2] Elevated cortisol levels can cause the body to activate the FAT Programs,[3] so just the act of being in SMART Mode can help you to turn off the FAT Programs (there's more about cortisol in the next section).

For now, however, the purpose is to develop the habit of having a SMART Mode session every day for at least ten minutes. In ten minutes, you can accomplish a lot. You can spend five minutes getting into SMART Mode (see chapter 5), and once you're in SMART Mode, you can spend five minutes practicing various visualizations.

Ideally, your SMART Mode sessions should be in the same location and at the same time of the day every day. It should be a place where noise or other people won't disturb you. Make sure you unplug the phone and tell the other members of your household that you don't want to be disturbed.

By far the best time of the day to have this SMART Mode session is first thing in the morning. In fact, the more of your life you can live in the morning the better. I strongly recommend that, if you're not doing so now, you find a way to carve out a block of time just for yourself when you first wake up. If you only need ten minutes for a SMART Mode session, it really only means going to sleep ten minutes earlier.

By having a SMART Mode session first thing in the morning, you can flush out all of the accumulated stress from the previous day. You start the day fresh, centered, and focused, so that any potentially stressful events that may occur in the coming day will be less likely to unbalance you.

After a full day, the evenings are often unproductive, passive hours. In the evenings, we are usually exhausted, and when we are exhausted, the only thing we can do is eat and be entertained. It's the exhausted, stressed-out evening hours where the majority of bingeing occurs.

If you don't have the visualization / SMART Mode session first thing in the morning, remember that whatever time of the day you do practice should be *the same time of the day every day and preferably in the same location.*

A Sample Ten-Minute SMART Mode Session

- Go to the room where you'll be practicing.
- Get into SMART Mode (five minutes—see chapter 5).
- Practice visualizing your ideal body (thirty seconds—see chapter 7).
- Practice one or two of the techniques found in chapter 6 for developing the ability to generate positive emotions automatically (two minutes).
- Visualize the rest of your day and how you would like it to unfold (thirty seconds).
- Then visualize the coming weeks, months, and even years, and see yourself living a happy, successful, and fulfilling life—and being in your ideal shape (thirty seconds).
- Finally, if appropriate, spend a moment asking for help and guidance with weight loss and life from a higher power, according to your beliefs (thirty seconds).

You will be amazed at how different you'll feel after ten short minutes. You'll feel calmer, and more centered and focused. You will experience a newfound sense of enthusiasm for life. Daily events that used to bother you will simply slide off you like water off a duck's back, and you'll have the energy to take on the world.

Just like strengthening a muscle, you'll get better at going into SMART Mode with practice. As a result, you'll get into SMART Mode more quickly, you'll go deeper, and the techniques will be much more effective.

The other benefit of this morning session is that it is a mechanism you can use for improving any aspect of your life you wish to improve. Once in SMART Mode, simply visualize the desired outcome, such as a promotion, moving to a new location, being happily married—whatever. *It's all within reach.*

By listening to the CD at night and having a morning visualization session, you now have two very powerful techniques to totally transform your body and any other aspect of your life that you desire.

NOTES

1. See "Stress" report, Well-Connected Website (Nidus Information Services, September 2001): http://www.well-connected.com/report.cgi/fr000031.html.

2. See A. Wilson, J. Davidson, and R. Jevning, "Adrenocortical Activity During Meditation," *Hormones and Behavior* 10, no. 1 (Society for Behavioral Neuroendocrinology, February 1978): 54–60.

3. See the Appendix (page 185) for more information on the relationship between elevated cortisol levels and the FAT Programs.

PART III

Physical Stresses that Activate the FAT Programs

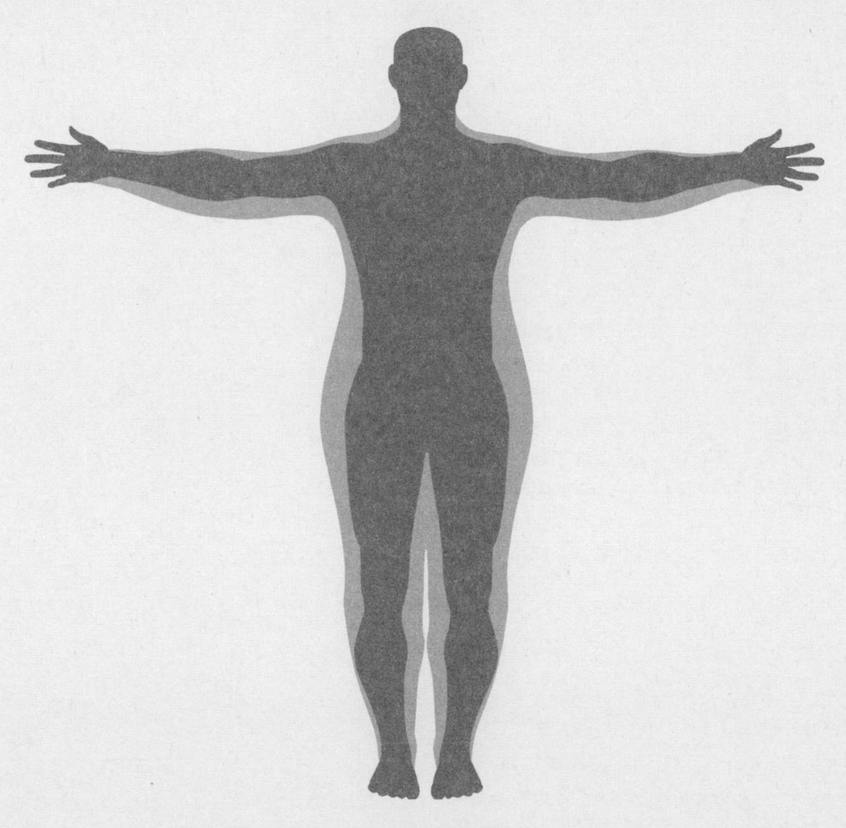

9

Why Diets Don't Work

Now that you understand the crucial importance of the mind-body connection to weight loss, let's turn our attention to some of the physical stresses that may be activating your Fat Programs and discuss what you can do about them. The number one physical stress that makes your body want to be fat is dieting.

Dieting—actively depriving yourself of certain foods—activates the FAT Programs. The stress of forcing yourself to eat less and of denying yourself the foods you're craving, day in and day out, causes hormonal and chemical changes in your body. These changes act as a signal to your brain that it's time to go into fat conservation mode (see the appendix on page 185 if you would like a more detailed explanation).

Dieting sends only one message to your brain: "There's not enough food. We'd better put every spare calorie we can into fat because we don't know where our next meal is coming from." In essence, dieting sends a famine message to your body that triggers the FAT Programs, and that's why diets don't work.

It's unlikely that anyone has ever told a person struggling with excess weight to *eat more*, but if you're starving yourself to try to lose weight, *that's exactly what I'm recommending you do*.

Diets all follow a similar pattern. By eliminating or severely restricting items from your diet, your body will, for a time, lose weight. You may lose weight quickly at first, but then the rate at which you lose weight will start to slow. Eventually, you stop losing weight altogether. You find yourself in the unfortunate position of having to restrict yourself, count calories, or follow unnatural eating schedules, not to lose weight, but to simply maintain your current level of body fat. You feel like you're running on a treadmill that just keeps going faster. The longer you go, the harder it gets.

From your body's perspective, you're now stuck in starvation mode; your appetite increases and it takes a lot more food before you feel full. Your taste buds become desensitized, and you start craving sweet and fatty foods. Your brain also sends a message to your thyroid to slow down your metabolism. This causes you to stop losing weight even though you are now eating less. Also, your body goes into perpetual fat storage mode: you become very efficient at storing fat and you lose the ability to burn it.

As a result, when dieting, you're hungry all the time and constantly fighting cravings. Then when you finally give in to your cravings, you gain the weight back very quickly because *all* those excess calories turn into fat. If you now go back to eating the way you used to, you'll get fatter on even fewer calories than before.

Many experts now concur that dieting can actually *make you fat*. Studies have shown that teenagers who diet are statistically three times more likely to be fat in five years time.[1] And I am sure that you, or someone you may know, has been on the "roller-coaster" of weight as a result of a string of unsuccessful diets. Why would this happen if dieting actually worked?

So why do so many people diet? People diet because they don't know any better. Conventional wisdom—what you may have learned as a child or growing up—strongly stands by the idea that eating less equals weighing less, and the only difference between a successful and unsuccessful dieter is will power. But the chemical evidence is clear beyond a shadow of a doubt: dieting doesn't work. Dieting makes your body *want* to be fat.

Diet-Free Weight Loss

If dieting doesn't work, what's the answer? Simple: eat more real foods!

What does this mean? Real foods are anything we ate prior to so-called civilization—before we learned how to "improve food" by processing it and packaging it to last forever. This includes live fruit, raw nuts and seeds, vegetables, salads (preferably organic), organic grass-fed meats, free-range chicken, and fish (see my website for Super Delicious / Super Nutritious recipes).

This is not to say that you have to eat these foods to the *exclusion* of others; you just have to *add* more of them to your current diet. Once you are nourishing your body, it will no longer want to be fat. As a result, your body will start to prefer real foods to the dead, processed, refined, artificial varieties we've become accustomed to eating.

Dieting is the act of forcing yourself to eat less, forcing yourself not to eat certain foods that you crave, or both. None of the three methods work, but adding foods that are missing and adding missing nutrients is easy and effective. My anti-diet strategy is to increase the body's desire to eat real foods while gradually eliminating the body's cravings for artificial and fake foods.

However, if you don't want to wait and you want to completely eradicate your cravings for any particular junk food instantly, please see chapter 18 to read about using visualization to kill food addictions.

It makes sense that, if certain foods don't attract you, or better yet, if they do repulse you, then avoiding them will take no effort. If someone told you that you had to live the rest of your life without eating cardboard or dirt or bugs you would say, "Big deal! So what?" It's no different with fake foods. Once your body understands that fake foods are starving or poisoning you, your body will start to reject them. And once your body rejects them, you're home free.

Also, don't convince yourself that a doughnut is a better snack than something like fruit, nuts, or seeds simply because it may have less calories. This is an illusion. If you eat foods that have no nutritional value, all you are doing is replenishing your sugar and fat stores, and you'll remain unsatisfied because you haven't nourished your body. Calories aren't everything.

The net result is you'll end up being hungry again a short time later. The more nutritious the food, the more you'll be satisfying your body. You'll be less hungry, and in the end, you'll consume fewer calories.

What We're Really Starving For

Even though we may have all the food in the world at our disposal today and we can be eating to our heart's content, we can still, nonetheless, be starving.

There are two fundamental reasons why we need to eat: (1) calories and (2) nutrients. A calorie literally means how much energy an item of food will provide your body, while a nutrient is a vitamin, mineral, fat, carbohydrate, or other essential building block that supports cellular health, integrity, or normal functioning. Most of the food we eat today has calories but very few nutrients; as a result, even though we may be eating more than enough calories, we are starving nutritionally.

Food isn't what it used to be. The so-called "food" we are eating today is drastically different from the food our ancestors ate. The foods our ancestors ate were mostly live, unprocessed foods like fruit, nuts, seeds, leafy greens, and freshly caught meat and fish. These types of foods have a full range of all the essential nutrients in a form that our bodies can digest and assimilate.

Much of the food we eat today is fattening, not because it contains too many calories but because the nutrients it contains are inadequate and unable to be assimilated. This is more specifically what I mean when I use the term "fake" foods. The nutrients in many modern foods are either scant, of poor quality, or in such an unnatural state that our bodies don't know what to do with them.

Comparing what our bodies are yearning for to what we're feeding them is like mining for diamonds. Your body has to sort through tons of material in order to find those few precious gems. Sure, there's tons of rubble and plenty of calories there, but the diamond nutrients that were once abundant aren't present anymore. Your body stays hungry in the hope of getting one or two precious nutrients, all the while storing away all the excess calories that come with them into your fat cells.

This is a key insight:

Your body will think it's starving and activate the FAT Programs, not only if there aren't enough calories, but also if there aren't enough essential nutrients.

Your body interprets a lack of essential nutrients as yet another form of famine. When we finally do eat things containing the nutrients our bodies are starving for on a daily basis, our bodies get the message: "OK. I'm not starving anymore. I don't need this fat anymore. It's safe to be thin now. Turn the FAT Programs off. NOW!"

NOTES

1. See "Teenage Dieters Are More Likely to be Overweight and Suffer from Eating Disorders in the Future," Medical News Today Website (April 14, 2006): http://www.medicalnewstoday.com/articles/41494.php.

10

The Essentials

It's very simple. Not all calories are equal. Not all fats are equal. Not all proteins are equal. Your body doesn't treat all sugars and starches the same way. Vitamins and minerals need to work together in the right combinations to work at all, and if the minerals are in the wrong form, you won't be able to use them. Chalk is full of calcium. But you could eat a ton of chalk and not get any calcium whatsoever. In the same way, milk is full of calcium, but when you pasteurize it, the chemical structure of the calcium changes. It becomes "denatured" and virtually unassimilable.

Just because you put it in your body doesn't mean that it ends up in your cells.

Starvation for essential nutrients may occur for many reasons, not all of them obvious.

We all need proteins, carbohydrates, and fats. If you're overweight, you might be thinking, "Isn't too much fat already one of my problems?" More likely, your problem is you're getting too little of the right *kind* of fat. You need to eat more of the correct types of fats, proteins, and carbohydrates.

If most of the foods you eat are processed and not live, you become chronically deficient in essential fatty acids, amino acids, and sugars. This chronic deficiency, just like any form of starvation, can activate the FAT Programs. Your body then stays hungry in the hope that you will eventually eat the nutrients you are starving for.

Fats, proteins, and carbohydrates are the big three—the things that our bodies need a lot of in order to function properly. Let's look at fats first.

Essential Fatty Acids

The most glaring and pervasive form of nutritional starvation we experience today is for essential fatty acids.

The term "essential" means that we have to have the nutrient *and* our bodies must get that nutrient from an outside source—just like a vitamin. Our bodies can manufacture certain types of fats (synthetic diamonds if you will), but we have no choice but to get essential fatty acids from the food we eat.

The main types of essential fatty acids that we need on a daily basis are omega-3 and omega-6 fatty acids.

Very few foods in our modern diet have omega-3s. There was a time when there was much less saturated fat in our diet and the ratio of omega-6 fatty acids to omega-3 fatty acids was one-to-one. Today the ratio of omega-6 fatty acids to omega-3 fatty acids is twenty-to-one. We now have proportionally twenty times more omega-6 fatty acids than omega-3 fatty acids. This unnatural imbalance causes inflammation, which is a major FAT Program activator.[1]

Countless scientific studies have shown that adding omega-3 fatty acids helps to switch off the FAT Programs.[2] In my opinion, it's next to impossible to lose weight on a consistent, permanent basis without having a sufficient, daily supply of quality omega-3 fatty acids.

Other studies have shown that omega-3 fatty acids are effective in treating all sorts of conditions.[3] To name a few:

- depression
- bipolar disorder

- heart disease
- type-2 diabetes
- inflammation
- aches and pains
- arthritis

The reason that we are lacking in omega-3s is that they're very easily corrupted. Too much exposure to heat, sunlight, and oxygen will destroy them as will most cooking and preservation methods—so any type of processed or packaged foods no longer contain viable omega-3 fatty acids. Most of the sources of fat we eat are from vegetable oils, meat, and dairy products. The majority of vegetable oils are mainly composed of processed, corrupted, unusable omega-6 fatty acids and contain an extremely detrimental form of fat called transfats. Meat and dairy products used to contain omega-3 fats, but now they are mostly saturated fats[4]—the result of feeding cows grain rather than grass.

We are so severely starving for omega-3 fatty acids that this is possibly the number one type of physical stress that triggers the FAT Programs.

So what's the solution? Don't go a single day without getting your essential fatty acids—especially omega-3.

How to Get More Uncorrupted Omega-3s into Your Diet

- **Flaxseed oil** is a very rich source of omega-3s. Use it in salads and salad dressings, as it is not a cooking oil. Flaxseed oil becomes rancid very easily when exposed to heat, sunlight, or oxygen. For this reason, you should keep the oil refrigerated for maximum effectiveness and use it only on food that is cold. Ground flaxseeds (linseeds) are excellent because they not only contain omega-3s but they also have protein and fiber. You can buy preground flaxseeds, but as soon as you grind them up, the oils start to become rancid. So it's best to buy the seeds whole and grind them fresh in a coffee grinder every morning. That's what I do. Then I sprinkle them on most of my food throughout the day. You can put them on almost anything—even dessert—for a nice nutty taste and texture.

- Eat more **fish**, especially coldwater fish, and fish caught in the wild as opposed to "farmed" or aqua-cultivated fish. And less cooking the better. If you deep fry fish, you are left with no semblance of usable omega-3s. As it is, you are lucky to retain about 30 percent of the oils, no matter how you cook it. Also, if the fish is farmed, the oil is higher in omega-6 fatty acids and lower in omega-3s.[5] Interestingly, when a 115-year-old Danish woman was asked what her secret was to such a long life, she said that she made it a point to have at least one piece of herring a day.
- Eat **organic meat and organic dairy** foods from grass-fed animals. If the animal is not grass-fed, then the fat is all *saturated fat*, not *essential fats*, so this only applies to grass-fed meat and dairy products.
- Use **omega-3-enriched eggs**. These are eggs that are produced by chickens that have been fed flaxseeds. Boiled eggs have more uncorrupted omega-3s than fried eggs because the temperature of boiling water is lower.

I recommend that in addition to eating more of these foods every day, you also supplement your diet with five to ten grams of omega-3 capsules. It sounds like a lot, but 10 grams of essential fat only translates to 100 calories of fat. That's less fat than what is contained in a small serving of potato chips. The difference here is that this extra fat is the kind your body is starving for.

You also need to have a good source of vitamin E when you are taking omega-3 fatty acids because it helps eliminate the toxic effect of eating corrupted or rancid oil.

One way or another, I get my omega-3s. I find a way. This has to be a daily thing—it's a must! It takes time to override the ill effects caused by years of being chronically starved for omega-3 fatty acids. In order to communicate to your body that omega-3s are abundant and that they will always be available, never miss a single day.

Frying Oils

When you heat oil to frying temperature, you usually destroy any of the beneficial properties of the oil. However, some oils are better than others for cooking. The best ones are organic butter, olive oil, and coconut oil. Coconut oil is a saturated fat, but it is a "medium-chain" saturated fat. Some researchers claim that these medium-chain saturated fats (MCSFs) are actually beneficial for weight loss because they speed up the metabolism.[6] I don't agree, but it is a fact that MSCFs can withstand high temperatures and not get corrupted, so whatever is beneficial about them will at least be preserved. Fats are just the first of the big three. Proteins are vital too.

Essential Amino Acids

Amino acids are the building blocks of protein. Proteins build nerves and muscle, and are essential to all bodily functions. We get protein from the foods we eat, and we disassemble the proteins to get the amino acids. It's like taking down a wall to get the bricks; we then use these bricks to build other proteins to suit our needs.

Although most of us eat plenty of protein, what you may not know is that the vast majority of the protein you eat may be unusable to your body. Just as heat and processing can destroy essential fatty acids, they can also destroy amino acids, rendering them useless as a source of protein. Most of the sources of protein we eat come from foods that are packaged or cooked. Therefore, even though we may be getting plenty of protein, our bodies may still be starving for it because the protein is corrupted or denatured. Your body can't use corrupted proteins because they are unassimilable.

Like everything else, it's not how much protein you are eating that's relevant but how much you are assimilating into the cells of your body. Corrupt proteins cannot be broken down properly. You could be eating 100 grams of protein a day, and out of the 100 grams, it's possible that as little as fifteen grams are usable. We have to do something with the leftovers, and what usually happens is that our bodies convert the remainder of the protein to sugar. This means it just becomes another source of empty calories that your body stores as fat.

Colostrum, the highly nutritious substance that comes out of a mother's breast for the first few weeks before the milk is produced, is said to be only 2 to 4 percent protein. At a time when humans are growing faster than at any other time in their lives, a time when they grow as much as 30 percent in a two-week period, they do so on a diet which consists of only 2 to 4 percent protein. We are able to do this because the protein is so highly assimilable.

So what's the solution to essential amino acid malnutrition? Eat more good, assimilable sources of protein:

- One of the most assimilable forms of protein is **whey protein**. You can buy whey protein powder at your health food store. I recommend the unsweetened, unflavored variety, preferably from sheep's or goat's milk, and organic. Unflavored whey protein has a creamy consistency and can be added to anything sweet or savory without compromising the taste. Try adding it to yogurt, creamy salad dressings, muesli, cereal, pancake and French toast batter, and any type of cake mix or bread dough. It also makes great protein shakes, fruit smoothies, and ice cream (see my website gabrielmethod.com/recipes for Super Delicious / Super Nutritious recipe suggestions).
- Other good sources of protein include **grass-fed organic meat**, **free-range chicken**, and **freshwater fish**. Also beneficial are **organic yogurts** and **white cheeses**, especially from goat's and sheep's milk. **Raw (not roasted) nuts and seeds** can also be good sources of protein.

How to Get the Most Out of Your Meat

- If you eat meat, the healthiest is grass-fed and organic.
- Meat is best digested when eaten by itself or with salad.
- Eat meat in a meal before the carbohydrates.
- Cook the meat less to avoid corrupting the proteins as much.

Picking the right fats and proteins is of paramount importance in weight loss, but don't ignore carbohydrates either. The right carbs are essential and the wrong ones can activate the FAT Programs.

Essential Sugars

Researchers have only recently discovered that, just as there are essential fatty acids and amino acids, there are also essential sugar compounds.[7] These essential sugars are important because they help your body build larger molecules called glycans.

Glycans help your immune system by binding to viruses and bacteria, making them harmless. They also help your cells to communicate with each other, particularly nerve and brain cells. A diet rich in unprocessed fruit and vegetables should give you all the essential sugars you need; not all of them are sweet or from sweet sources. For example:

- Fucose—mushrooms and seeds
- Xylose—barley and yeast
- Mannose—broccoli, cabbage, and seeds

Sugars, essential or otherwise, are one form of carbohydrate—the principle form of energy besides fat. The real issue as far as carbohydrates are concerned is what I call "dead" carbohydrates, especially processed grains, starches, and refined sugar. These carbohydrates do not have any usable essential nutrients. The more we eat of them, the more we starve. Dead carbohydrates are just empty calories that get stored in our fat cells. They also trick our bodies hormonally into activating the FAT Programs.[8] The worst forms of dead carbohydrates are processed bread and other wheat products, and table sugar.

Fruit, on the other hand, which is also a source of carbohydrates, is invaluable for effectively eliminating many of the most common forms of starvation that make your body want to be fat.

All live fruit has essential sugars. Most fruit helps to regulate blood sugar. Some fruit, like berries, are considered one of the greatest sources of antioxidants around. Antioxidants are essential for neutralizing dangerous, unstable chemical compounds in the body that can damage cells and DNA.

Fruit also has protein and, although it has a smaller amount than most foods that are traditionally eaten for their protein content, the protein in live fruit is uncorrupted and contains the digestive enzymes required to facilitate easy assimilation. It's not so much the quantity of protein that matters but how much of it can be assimilated.

Fruit causes the blood to become more alkaline, which is also very important for the removal of toxins. Most of the food we eat, such as sugar, starches, meat, and grains, are all acid producing. An acid environment is where most diseases thrive. The action of trying to counteract the acid environment that these foods cause is a chronic source of stress that can activate the FAT Programs. The body is often forced to extract calcium from our bones and teeth to neutralize acid waste. This causes the body to become depleted of calcium, and calcium, we are just finding out, is truly essential for weight loss.[9]

Make an Informed Choice

I just talked about processed, refined, conventionally-farmed, "dead" carbs and how things like bread, cereal, pasta, sugar, potatoes, and processed foods can be among your biggest enemies. Eat them as long as your body still craves them because eventually the cravings will go away. However, in the meantime, any time you are presented with a choice between eating a meal that has these foods or one that doesn't, choose the one that doesn't. *Only do this if you are genuinely indifferent to the choice.* Choosing to eat healthier food when you truly don't care about other alternatives is a perfect opportunity to speed things along.

For example, if you are eating out and there's a choice between lasagna with mashed potatoes and a side order of macaroni and cheese, or almond-crusted, grilled chicken with field greens drizzled in honey-balsamic vinegar dressing and young asparagus spears in hollandaise sauce, go with the chicken.

The worst time to eat dead carbs is late at night because they'll keep your body in fat storage mode[10] all night. That means you will be making fat all night. If you eat dead carbs for breakfast or lunch, you have a better chance of actually using the sugar, instead of storing it in your fat cells. The best way to eat dead carbs is with some source of essential fat, protein, fiber, or all three. Eat the fat, protein, and fiber before the dead carbs and it will slow down the rate at which the sugar enters your blood stream. If you're out to dinner, it's better to have the bread after you have eaten your appetizer or after you have had some of your meal. Also, pick the most whole-grain, seedy, nutty bread that you can get, as this has more fiber, essential fats, and protein.

Here is a list of different types of breads, in order of preference:

1. Sprouted grain breads: These are usually found in the refrigerated foods section of your health food store. They are made of sprouted grains instead of milled grains, and they are very good for you. Some of them taste excellent, but they don't really taste like the breads you may be used to. You can cut slices off and toast them, and they go well with almond butter and banana slices. They make a great sandwich with sprouts, avocado, chicken, mustard, and other condiments and toppings. You can also use them for French toast.

2. Homemade breads: Buy organic whole grains from your health food store and grind them into flour with a coffee grinder. You can then use this flour with other ingredients in a homemade bread maker. Experiment with different grains, nuts, seeds, and fruits, and note that it is important to make the bread as soon as you grind the grain into flour.

3. Store-bought organic, wheat-free, and gluten-free bread: These are breads made out of grains such as spelt and rice and specifically say that they are gluten free. Gluten is a non-nutritious, gluey substance in bread that interferes with your body's ability to digest and assimilate nutrients.

4. Organic wheat-free bread: These are breads made of organic grains like spelt, rice, rye, and oats.

5. Organic whole wheat bread: This is bread made from organic whole wheat.

Once you fall below this standard to conventionally-farmed wheat bread, whether whole wheat or not, you are eating something that is substantially worse for you. Conventionally-farmed grains have over twenty different pesticides, stabilizers, preservatives, and fungicides. They are stripped of all nutrients, and the toxic by-products block your body's ability to absorb other nutrients from other foods.[11]

There is one other major advantage to eating live organic fruits and vegetables: they have a quality that only live organic food has. It's a quality lacking in the overcooked, over processed, artificially flavored, dead foods that make up the majority of our modern day diet. That quality is *vitality*.

NOTES

1. See the appendix (page 185) for how proinflammatory cytokines can activate the FAT Programs.

2. For more on how omega-3 fatty acids increase insulin sensitivity and reverse hyperinsulinemia, see R. Rosedale, MD, "Insulin and Its Metabolic Effects," Mercola.com Newsletter (July 2001): http://articles.mercola.com/sites/articles/archive/2001/07/14/insulin-part-one.aspx. And for a discussion on how omega-3 fatty acids reduce inflammation and proinflammatory cytokines," see B. Holub, "Clinical Nutrition 4: Omega-3 Fatty Acids and Cardio Vascular Care," *Canadian Medical Associaton Journal* 166, no. 5 (Canadian Medical Association, March 5, 2002): 608–615; A. Sher, C. Serhan, F. Bianchini, J. Aliberti, M. Arita, N. Chiang, N. Petasis, R. Yang, and S. Hong, "Stereochemical Assignment, Anti-inflammatory Properties, and Receptor for the Omega-3 Lipid Mediator Resolvin E1," *The Journal of Experimental Medicine* 201, no. 5 (Rockefeller University Press, March 7, 2005): 713–722; and L. G. Cleland,

M. J. James, et al., "The Role of Fish Oils in the Treatment of Rheumatoid Arthritis," *Drugs* 63, no. 9 (Adis, 2003): 845–853. And see the appendix (page 185) for the relationship between insulin resistance, elevated triglycerides, inflammation and the FAT Programs.

3. See L. Arab, "Biomarkers of Fat and Fatty Acid Intake," *The Journal of Nutrition* 133, no. 3 (American Society for Nutrition, March 2003): 925S–932S; I. Mustafa and M. M. Berger, "Metabolic and Nutritional Support in Acute Cardiac Failure," *Current Opinion in Clinical Nutrition Metabolic Care* 6, no. 2 (Lippincott Williams & Wilkins, March 2003): 195–201; D. Bhatnagar and P. Durrington, "Omega-3 Fatty Acids: Their Role in the Prevention and Treatment of Atherosclerosis-Related Risk Factors and Complications," *International Journal of Clinical Practice* 57, no. 4 (Blackwell Publishing, May 2003): 305–314; R. R. Brenner, "Hormonal Modulation of Delta6 and Delta5 Desaturases: Case of Diabetes," *Prostaglandins, Leukotrienes Essential Fatty Acids* 68, no. 2 (Elsevier, February 2003): 151–162; P. C. Calder, "Long-Chain N-3 Fatty Acids and Inflammation: Potential Application in Surgical and Trauma Patients," *Brazilian Journal of Medical and Biological Research* 36, no. 4 (2003): 433–446; S. J. Yeh and W. J. Chen, "Effects of Fish Oil in Parenteral Nutrition," *Nutrition* 19, no. 3 (Elsevier, March 2003): 275–279; A. Colin, J. Reggers, et al., "Lipids, Depression and Suicide," *Encephale* 29, no. 1 (Elsevier, Jan.–Feb. 2003): 49–58; M. Haag, "Essential Fatty Acids and the Brain," *Canadian Journal of Psychiatry* 48, no. 3 (Canadian Psychiatric Association, April 2003): 195–203; S. Harris, Y. Park, et al., "Cardiovascular Disease and Long-Chain Omega-3 Fatty Acids," *Current Opinion in Lipidololgy* 14, no. 1 (Lippincott Williams & Wilkins, February 2003): 9–14; C. Hennekens and J. Skerrett, "Consumption of Fish and Fish Oils and Decreased Risk of Stroke," *Preventive Cardiology* 6, no. 1 (American Society for Preventive Cardiology, 2003): 38–41; and L. Spector and M. Surette, "Diet and Asthma: Has the Role of Dietary Lipids Been Overlooked in the Management of Asthma?" *Annals of Allergy, Asthma, and Immunology* 90, no. 4 (American College of Allergy, Asthma & Immunology, April 2003): 371–378, 421.

4. See R. Rosedale, *The Rosedale Diet* (New York: Harper Collins, 2004).

5. See J. Rubin, *The Maker's Diet* (New York: Penguin, 2004).

6. See http://www.mercola.com/products/coconut_oil.htm for more on coconut oil as a smart cooking alternative.

7. See J. Thompson, "Essential 8," The Health Sciences Institute Website (October 14, 2004): http://www.hsibaltimore.com/ealerts/ea200410/ea20041014.html.

8. Eating a diet high in processed grains and refined sugars can lead to leptin and insulin resistance. For more on this, see R. Rosedale, "Insulin and Its Metabolic Effects," Mercola.com Newsletter (July 2001): http://articles.mercola.com/sites/articles/archive/2001/07/14/insulin-part-one.aspx; and R. Rosedale, *The Rosedale Diet* (New York: Harper Collins, 2004).

9. See J. Yanovski and S. Parikhand, "Calcium Intake and Adiposity," *American Journal of Clinical Nutrition* 77, no. 2 (February 2003): 281–287.

10. See J. Allbritin, "Wheaty Indiscretions: What Happens to Wheat, from Seed to Storage," *Wise Traditions in Food, Farming, and the Healing Arts* 4, no. 1 (Weston A. Price Foundation, Spring 2003).

11. Ibid.

11

Vitality: The Zero-Calorie Essential Nutrient

There is another component to food that our bodies require, other than calories, protein, fats, carbohydrates, and various chemical nutrients, and that's the life force in the food itself. When we are eating "live," biologically active food, we are assimilating the life force of that food.

Cultures around the world and throughout history have acknowledged that a subtle energy surrounds, permeates, and animates all living things. This energy enables life and translates thought into movement. It allows the autonomic nervous system to keep the heart beating and the blood circulating. When this energy is gone, the connection is severed and death results. The body then just becomes a highly organized structure of decomposing chemicals.

Vital energy has had many names throughout history—Ch'i/Ki/Qi, Prana, Shakti, life force, subtle energy, and more recently, orgone, and biophotons, to name just a few. In our own bodies this energy travels along particular paths, known as acupuncture meridians in Chinese medicine. They are also referred to as *nadis* in Indian Ayurvedic medicine.

We can be devitalized, not only because we don't have enough life force in our bodies but also because these energy channels, or meridians, can get blocked. Chinese medicine believes that stress, toxins, low-energy thinking, and negative emotions cause blockages in the flow of subtle energy, and that these blockages are the root cause of all sicknesses and depression. Disease, according to Chinese doctors, manifests first as an energy blockage before it materializes as a physical ailment.

Blocked energy stagnates, and stagnation is devitalization. Just as a stagnant puddle of water is less healthy to drink than a flowing stream, the stagnant energy in our bodies is less healthy than flowing energy.

Devitalization Is the Kiss of Death for Weight Loss

Devitalization causes stress, activates the FAT Programs,[1] and makes us perpetually hungry and tired. Because we are exhausted all of the time, we crave sugar to boost our energy. As a result, we end up eating junk food just to get through the day. We also get upset more easily and we become more prone to low-energy negative thinking. This creates more stress, more negative emotions, more energy blockages, and more devitalization—a vicious cycle indeed.

You can unblock energy pathways by reducing stress, negative thinking, and negative emotions—all things we talked about in the previous section. You can also replenish this energy by spending more time in nature.

In the Space Age world, we very rarely interact with the elements in our natural environment. There is vitality everywhere in nature; sunlight, fresh air, fresh water, earth, trees, mountains, and grass all have their own energy that we absorb when we are in their presence. Up until very recently, we spent most of our time outdoors, interacting with and absorbing this energy. Now we spend most of our time indoors, cut off from the nourishing vitality of nature and thus remain devitalized—starving for vitality.

You can also replenish this particular energy by eating more live and vibrant foods. At the moment, nutritionists and experts focus on the things that they are certain exist, such as calories, carbohydrates, proteins, fats, vitamins, minerals, antioxidants, phytonutrients, and the like. But these are all just chemicals—

essential, yes, but the picture is incomplete. Our mainstream science doesn't recognize this vital energy as an essential element in the food we eat for one simple reason: we currently have no instruments to identify it, quantify it, or to track its movement. Then again, we didn't know bacteria existed until we invented the microscope, or that radio waves existed until we invented the receiver.

Humans are infinitely more complex and valuable than just the chemicals that make up our bodies, and live food is infinitely more nutritious than just its chemical composition. Today, nearly all of our foods are canned, packaged, processed, or cooked and, therefore, dead and devitalized. The trend of eating more dead food and less live food has been increasing at an exponential rate over the last fifty years—at roughly the same rate that obesity has been increasing.

Studies are coming out all the time that validate the notion that what our bodies are really craving from food is this invisible, energetic component. Of particular interest is the technique of counting photon emissions. Every living organism emits biophotons or low-level luminescence (light with a wavelength between 200 and 800 nanometers). This light energy is thought to be stored in DNA during photosynthesis and is transmitted continuously by the cell.

Some researchers have concluded that the higher the level of light energy a cell emits from the food we eat, the greater the value. This light energy comes from the sun, and the more sunlight that can be stored at a cellular level, the greater the potential for the transfer of that energy to the individual who consumes it.[2]

The Vitamin D Connection

There is mounting evidence that eating live foods and spending time in the sun turns off the FAT Programs, and this evidence relates to vitamin D. Vitamin D, we are now just discovering, is essential for turning off the FAT Programs. There is growing statistical evidence that suggests that obesity may be linked to vitamin D deficiency,[3] and the best source of vitamin D is sunlight.

Studies have found that raw food vegans, people who eat a diet of only live foods, have higher levels of vitamin D than other people.[4] This is incredible when you consider that it was once believed that eating meat was the only way to get vitamin D. One possible explanation for this is that live foods contain the same energetic component that sunlight does, and we convert this subtle energy into vitamin D—just like we do with sunlight. Please note, though, that I am not suggesting that you become a live-food vegan or a sun worshipper; I *am* suggesting that you place more value on live foods by adding them to your diet whenever possible, and that you get sun in the safest way possible.

When we eat live foods, we assimilate life. Eating dead foods only brings us closer to death. How many calories we need in a day is not the question we should be asking ourselves. The real questions are: How much vitality do we need in a day, and how can we get this vitality?

Calories and vitality have nothing to do with each other. We can eat five thousand calories in a day, but if we have not gotten our daily dose of vitality, we can still feel hungry. When we get the necessary vitality our bodies are starving for in a few supercharged choice calories, we'll feel completely satisfied. It's this vitality that makes us feel completely satisfied and not the short-term, addictive experience of eating dead, processed chemicals.

Every time we discover a new essential component in food, we find that it's only present in live foods; processing food either destroys that component or completely strips it out. Someone usually figures out how to bottle and market an expensive supplement in order to replace this item, but simply eating more live food would give us all the benefits and more.

Stripping the essential nutrients from the foods we eat and then having someone sell them back to us piece by piece in tablet form is sad and ironic. I wonder if, when the mainstream accepts the validity of life force and acknowledges its essential role in our diet, someone is going to try to sell it to us in tablet form?

So what's the solution to vitality malnutrition?

Foods that contain the most vitality are live, preferably organic, in season, and locally grown. Foods with live chlorophyll have the most vitality. (Chlorophyll is the substance in plants that converts sunlight into nutrients.) All types of salads and sprouts are great—the greener the better! The food with the most vitality and live chlorophyll is fresh-squeezed wheatgrass juice (see page 130 for more on wheatgrass juice).

You don't only get vitality from eating live foods; spend a few quiet minutes a day in nature. I know this isn't always convenient if you live in a city. But perhaps you can make it a point to go to a nearby park on a break or at least spend some time out in the sun. When I lived in New York City, I would go entire winters without seeing the sun (I went to work before it was light and came home after dark). It was also very rare for me to be around any trees or grass. My body was starving for nature, and this was a major contributing factor to my problem with obesity.

You can also absorb vitality directly from the sun.

The following is an easy technique that you can use to gain and assimilate more vitality directly from sunlight. This technique is based on five-thousand-year-old Chinese Taoist Chi Kung techniques. It may sound strange, and—by all means—if it feels funny to you, skip it. But I can tell you that it really works (don't knock it till you try it). It's quick, easy to perform, and extremely effective.

Technique for Vitality—Eating the Sun

- Stand up, preferably outside, with bare feet on the grass if that's possible or comfortable for you. Face the sun with your eyes closed and your palms out, and let the sun bathe your face, hands, and body.
- Focus your attention around your forehead, and visualize breathing the sunlight into your forehead. Feel that

your brain is being bathed with sunlight. Imagine that you're literally breathing sunlight into your forehead.

- Just remain like this for a minute or so and continue to breathe the sunlight into your forehead.
- Now open your mouth, and swallow a gulp of air and sunlight into your stomach. Then, while holding your breath, face your palms downward and lightly tense your arms, your abdomen, your buttocks, and your legs. Imagine that the energy of the sun is being absorbed into your bones, your muscles, and your lower back.
- Remain in this position for a moment or two. Feel the sunlight penetrating into the core of your bones and being stored there.
- Now exhale and relax for a moment. At that point, take another gulp of air and sun, and repeat. You can repeat this process as many times as you like. I usually do it three or four times.
- Then relax and enjoy the sun on your face for a little while longer.

If you feel self-conscious doing this exercise in public, sit on a more private park bench in the sun. Occasionally pretend to yawn and, while doing so, swallow some sunlight. Lightly tense your muscles, and imagine the vitality being absorbed into your bones. Or simply sit there and let the sun bathe your forehead. Even *this* will do a lot. There is very strong evidence that sunlight can help turn the FAT Programs off.[5]

Ideal Body Visualization While Eating the Sun

After completing the exercise, simply stand in the sunlight and imagine you are in the ideal shape that you'd like to be. This whole exercise should take no more than two to five minutes to perform.

Getting essential nutrients and vital energy is one part of the equation. But no matter how fresh and nutritious the food is, if we are unable to digest it properly and the nutrients are not entering the cells of our bodies, we can still be starving.

NOTES

1. Certain stress responses can cause elevated levels of cortisol and proinflammatory cytokines, which can lead to resistance of both insulin and leptins. For more on this, see C. Kristo, K. Godang, J. Bollerslev, P. Aukrust, and T. Ueland, "Interleukin-1 Receptor Antagonist is Associated with Fat Distribution in Endogenous Cushing's Syndrome: A Longitudinal Study," *The Journal of Clinical Endocrinology and Metabolism* 88, no. 4 (The Endocrine Society, 2003): 1492–1496; C. Kalhan, J. Challier, J. Friedman, J. Kirwan, J. Lepercq, L. Huston-Presley, P. Catalano, and S. Hauguel-De Mouzon, "TNF-alpha Is a Predictor of Insulin Resistance in Human Pregnancy," *Diabetes* 51, no. 7 (American Diabetes Association, July 2002): 2207–2213; I. Elenkov and P. Chrousos, "Stress Hormones, Proinflammatory and Anti-inflammatory Cytokines, and Autoimmunity," *Annals of the New York Academy of Sciences* 966 (June 2002): 290–303; and see the appendix (page 185) for the relationship between proinflammatory cytokines and the FAT Programs.

2. See J. Mercola, "McDonald's and Biophoton Deficiency," Mercola.com Newletter (August 21, 2002): http://articles.mercola.com/sites/articles/archive/2002/08/21/biophoton.aspx.

3. See J. Mercola, "Breakthough Updates You Need to Know On Vitamin D," Mercola.com Newsletter (February 23, 2002): http://articles.mercola.com/sites/articles/archive/2002/02/23/vitamin-d-part-five.aspx; A. Zittermann, R. Koerfer, and S. Schleithoff, "Putting Cardiovascular Disease and Vitamin D Insufficiency Into Perspective," *British Journal of Nutrition* 94, no. 4 (Cambridge University Press, October 2005): 483–492; and the appendix (page 185) for the relationship between proinflammatory cytokines and the FAT Programs.

4. See D. Villareal, J. Holloszy, J. Shew, and L. Fontana, "Low Bone Mass in Subjects on a Long-term Raw Vegetarian Diet," *Archives of Internal Medicine* 165, no. 6 (American Medical Association, March 28, 2005): 684–689.

5. For more on how sunlight increases melanocortin levels and the potential increase in the brain's leptin sensitivity, see M. Matheny, N. Tumer, P. J. Scarpace, S. Zolotukhin, and Y. Zhang, "Leptin-Induced Leptin-Resistant Rats Exhibit Enhanced Response to the Melanocortin Agonist MT II," *Neuropharmacology* 45, no. 2 (Elsevier, August 2003): 211–219; C. Kenny, C. Lee, C. Streamson, J. Elmquist, J. McMinn, N. Balthasar, R. Coppari, R. McGovern, S. Lui, and V. Tang, "Leptin Receptor Signaling in POMC Neurons Is Required for Normal Body Weight Homeostasis," *Neuron* 42, no. 6 (Elsevier, June 24, 2004): 963–991; D. Clegg, D. Drazen, and R. Seeley, "The Critical Role of the Melanocortin System in the Control of Energy Balance," *Annual Review of Nutrition* 24 (July 2004): 133–149; and the appendix for the relationship between leptin resistance and the FAT Programs.

12

It Doesn't Count Unless It Enters Your Cells

Even if we get all the nutrients our bodies are starving for, it still doesn't mean that we are nourishing our bodies. We can't necessarily make the assumption that what we put in our mouth will ultimately end up in our cells. After we eat something, there are three hurdles that we have to cross before the food ends up nourishing our bodies:

- We have to digest our food—break it down into simpler units that our bodies can then use as raw materials.
- We have to be able to transport the raw materials to the cells of our bodies.
- Once we have transported the nutrients to the cells, they have to be able to enter the cells.

Transporting the nutrients from the digestive tract and then creating an internal environment that makes it easy for the cells to absorb the nutrients is assimilation—the final leg of the digestion process. If this doesn't happen, we are simply not nourishing our bodies and, therefore, we continue to starve.

Enzymes and Digestion

One of the reasons that our ability to digest and assimilate nutrients is compromised is that we are deficient in digestive enzymes.

An enzyme is a specific type of protein that helps speed up chemical reactions; they are the workhorses of all life on Earth. Where there is life, there are enzymes doing some sort of work. And there are thousands of different kinds of enzymes in our bodies performing specific functions, such as facilitating physical movement or circulation, or fighting off toxins. The role of digestive enzymes is to break down foods into their basic nutritional components, thus allowing us to assimilate those nutrients. When we are deficient in digestive enzymes, we can't effectively extract the nutrients from the foods we eat. Consequently, it requires larger quantities of food to nourish our bodies because we are getting less real nutrition from our food.

There's a strong link between a lack of digestive enzymes and obesity,[1] and here are several reasons why we might be deficient:

- **Processing:** We have destroyed the enzymes in our food or made them unavailable. Live, biologically active foods contain digestive enzymes; it's these enzymes that cause a fruit or vegetable to ripen. When we eat foods that contain live, active enzymes, our bodies use these enzymes in conjunction with the body's enzymes to ensure the most complete digestion possible. However, heating and processing foods destroys the digestive enzymes in the foods themselves, forcing our bodies to produce more of their own—if our bodies are able.
- **Modern farming methods:** Pesticides, herbicides, chemical fertilizers, and irradiation lower the amount of biologically active digestive enzymes in food. Nearly all the food we eat today is either completely devoid of, or severely lacking in, live digestive enzymes. As a result, the body is forced to rely solely on its own ability to produce the enzymes necessary for digestion. This places undue stress on our pancreas, which produces digestive enzymes, and to add insult to injury, other systems of our body compete for these enzymes. The immune system, for example, uses enzymes to digest foreign bodies that it encounters in our

blood streams. This combination—no digestive enzymes in our food and the demands from our immune system for the enzymes that our bodies must manufacture—leaves us chronically deficient in digestive enzymes.

- **Temperature:** Besides the fact that cooking foods destroys biologically active digestive enzymes, when we eat foods that are hotter than our body temperature, our body's digestive enzymes become inactive. Our enzymes were designed to be active at or around our body temperature. Hot foods are usually eaten at temperatures much hotter than our body temperature, resulting in a digestive quandary of toxic decay in our intestines and a need for much more food to get the nutrients we require.
- **Mental and emotional stress:** Stress diverts the body's energy and blood flow away from digestion, lowering the body's effectiveness at producing digestive enzymes. Digestion is less complete when we are in a state of chronic stress.

Good Bacteria, Microbes, and Digestion

Another reason our digestion and assimilation is compromised is because our intestines are lacking in friendly bacteria and digestive microorganisms. Many years ago, the soil in which our food was grown was rich in plant-based microbes that are essential for effective digestion and assimilation of nutrients, as well as the removal of toxic waste in our digestive tracts. Pesticides, herbicides, and fertilizers kill these bacteria. Over-farming drains the soil of nutrients and bacteria without effectively replenishing them. We then destroy the remaining beneficial microorganisms with cooking and processing.

Antibiotics and chlorinated water destroy the microorganisms and friendly bacteria in our digestive tracts too. Because the foods have been stripped of beneficial bacteria, we never get a chance to replenish them. As a result, our stomachs and intestines get repopulated with unhealthy bacteria and fungi like yeast and candida instead. These types of fungi cause wheat and sugar cravings to satisfy their own food requirements. Not only are we severely inhibiting our ability to digest and assimilate nutrients, we are getting unnecessary junk food cravings as well. After finishing a course of antibiotics, for example, you should take large doses of probiotics to replenish your intestinal tract with friendly bacteria. Otherwise, your intestines will be repopulated with yeast, fungus, parasites, and unfriendly bacteria.

Food Combining and Digestion

The diet our ancestors ate prior to the agricultural revolution did not have any grains or dairy products. Combining grains and dairy products with meat products causes another digestive hurdle. Meat is digested in an extremely acidic environment in our stomachs; grains, starches, and dairy foods require a more alkaline medium. If we eat both at the same time, neither the meat nor the starches get properly digested.

It's best to eat meat and live food before grains and dairy because if you do you'll be able to digest both better. It's also preferable to eat grains after meat in order to slow down the rate at which the sugar from the grains is released into your blood stream. Having sugar enter you're blood stream slowly is truly crucial for weight loss.

Assimilation

Whatever nutrients do get extracted from the food we eat need to be able to travel freely through the blood stream to all the cells that require them. If our circulation is impaired because of blockages in our circulatory system, many cells will never be properly nourished.

Once the nutrients travel to the cells, they have to be able to enter them. When the FAT Programs are on, the cells become resistant to the effects of the hormone insulin.[2] Although many people are aware of the role of insulin in regulating blood sugar, one of insulin's other roles is to allow certain nutrients to enter cells. When the FAT Programs are on, many cells become less responsive to insulin. Nutrients cannot enter the cell, and as a result, the cell cannot be properly nourished (see the appendix on page 185).

Magnesium, for example, is one element that requires insulin to enter your cells.[3] If the cells aren't listening to insulin, you can take all the magnesium supplements you want to but you'll still remain deficient.

Being deficient in magnesium causes chronic exhaustion and chronic stress,[4] and this creates a vicious cycle. The chronic starvation for magnesium keeps the FAT Programs on, which then makes the cells stop listening to insulin even more, and that only makes it harder for magnesium and other vital nutrients to enter the cells. Eating a modern diet of processed foods wreaks havoc on the body's ability to digest and assimilate nutrients. If only a small percentage of the food we eat ends up nourishing our bodies, it requires much more food to get the job done. Couple this with the fact that the foods we eat have very little nourishment to begin with, and it's easy to see why so many of us are stuck in a state of chronic nutritional deprivation.

Periodontal Disease

There's mounting evidence to link the pathogens in the mouth from periodontal disease with the FAT Programs.[5] It may be no coincidence that a very large percentage of obese individuals also suffer from this ailment. These pathogens ultimately spread to our digestive track, killing our beneficial bacteria and compromising our absorption of nutrients. It's a good idea to get your teeth cleaned once a month for the first six months of your transformation. Also try to take good care of your teeth by brushing and flossing frequently. There are now also toothpastes available that have probiotics in them. I highly recommend using this sort of toothpaste, as this will help fight off pathogens and improve the positive bacteria culture of the mouth (please refer to my website gabrielmethod.com for recommended toothpastes).

Once you start naturally choosing foods that are healthier, gum disease should not trouble you as much, or at all. For the first six months, however, it's a good idea to be extra vigilant about your oral health.

So, What's the Solution?

All live, organic foods have digestive enzymes. If it is organic, it will also have digestive microbes. While dairy foods are not great, yogurt and kefir, a fermented, enzyme-rich milk drink, are good sources of beneficial bacteria. Yogurt, kefir, and, for that matter, all dairy products are much more effective when they are organic. Sheep's milk and goat's milk products are much easier to digest than those produced from cow's milk. Fermented foods, such as nutritional yeast and tempeh, are also rich in digestive enzymes.

I also recommend taking digestive enzymes and probiotic supplements every day. I don't believe in taking too many supplements, but I think digestive enzymes and probiotics are a must.

Digestive enzyme supplements are capsules or powders that contain the same digestive enzymes that our bodies produce. The best ones are derived from plant sources, not animal ones, because plant-based enzymes work within a wider pH range. You can take the capsules with meals, and you should try to take them at least once a day. A good thing to do is to make a habit of having them with your breakfast every day (we'll talk about how to make all of these suggestions habits at the end of book). You can also open the capsules and sprinkle them directly onto your food. This will give the enzymes a chance to predigest the food before you have eaten it.

Probiotics are capsules and powders that are a combination of beneficial bacteria and digestive microbes. Probiotics can also turn off FAT Programs by decreasing the amount of pro-inflammatory cytokines.[6] Try to find a probiotic that has a large assortment of bacteria and digestive microbes too. Digestive microbes are sometimes called homeostatic soil organisms (HSOs), or soil-based organisms (SBOs).[7] Probiotics should be taken on an empty stomach first thing in the morning. In addition, please make sure to take probiotics morning and evening for at least four weeks after taking antibiotics.

NOTES

1. See J. Thompson, "Chew On This," The Health Sciences Institute Website (December 12, 2003): http://www.hsibaltimore.com/ealerts/ea200312/ea20031204.html.

2. See the appendix (page 185) for the relationship between insulin resistance and the FAT Programs.

3. See R. Rosedale, "Insulin and Its Metabolic Effects," Mercola.com Newsletter (July 2001): http://articles.mercola.com/sites/articles/archive/2001/07/14/insulin-part-one.aspx.

4. Ibid.

5. See A. Ho, F. Nishimura, R. Genco, S. Grossi, and Y. Murayama, "A Proposed Model Linking Inflammation to Obesity, Diabetes, and Periodontal Infections," *Journal of Periodontology* 76, no. 11-s (American Academy of Periodontology, November 2005): 2075–2084.

6. See the appendix (page 185) for the relationship between proinflammatory cytokines and the FAT Programs.

7. See R. Rubin, *The Maker's Diet* (New York: Penguin, 2004).

13

Other Forms of Starvation

Chronic Dehydration—Starving for Water

Water covers over 70 percent of the planet, and our bodies are supposed to be made up of at least 70 percent water as well. Water is essential for life. Most of us would only be able to survive three days without water before dying of thirst.

It's estimated that as much as 75 to 80 percent of the population is in a state of chronic dehydration,[1] and chronic dehydration is stress that activates the FAT Programs. We often mistake dehydration for hunger, so many times we actually eat because we are thirsty. Dehydration also frequently manifests as a craving for sweets and soft drinks—the very things we should avoid when losing weight.

All dietary experts recommend drinking lots of water, and most agree that you should have a minimum of eight glasses of water a day. Some experts believe you should drink one ounce of water a day for every 2.2 pounds of body weight. That means that if you weigh 176 pounds you should drink eighty ounces of water, or ten glasses, a day.

Drinking water before a meal is effective in reducing your appetite; I usually drink two glasses before each meal. Most of the time, people eat when they are actually thirsty, so you have to learn how to identify thirst. And dehydration usually causes hunger, not thirst, because there was once a time when nearly all of our food contained water. Therefore, our bodies are programmed to see food as a source of water, sending a hunger message when we are really thirsty. The majority of our food today does not have much water at all. How much water is there in fried fish and chips, or peanut butter and crackers? We end up eating because we are dehydrated, and yet we are still starved for water.

Because there is less water in the food we eat, we need to drink more than ever. We also need more water these days because water helps eliminate toxins. There are literally thousands of toxins that we expose our bodies to today that did not exist in prehistoric times.

Learning how to identify the difference between hunger and thirst is essential. This is a lesson that has taken me years to learn, and I often have to relearn it. However, now that I have had a lot of practice in distinguishing between hunger and thirst, I have to say that there are times when I am amazed at how much water my body wants.

I also notice that my body becomes thirstier when it wants to burn fat. The process of losing weight requires more water to help you flush out the waste products that accumulate in the blood stream from the fat burning process.

As a general rule of thumb, until you become good at differentiating dehydration from hunger, especially if you eat a conventional modern diet, you are most likely to be thirsty. This is not to say that you may not be hungry as well, but you are almost certainly chronically dehydrated. If you don't give your body the water it needs, it will just stay hungry and cause you to eat unnecessarily.

Drinking water at night is extremely beneficial for suppressing nighttime hunger. A University of Washington study found that drinking water at night eliminated nighttime hunger pangs in 100 percent of the subject's tested.[2] I can't emphasize strongly enough the importance of drinking lots of water at night.

Water is best when filtered and free of chemical additives, and preferably from an unpolluted source. Adding lemon helps to detoxify the body, and I recommend avoiding tap water. Chlorinated water, such as tap water, kills the friendly bacteria in the stomach.

So what's the solution to chronic dehydration?

Drink two glasses of water first thing in the morning, a glass of water before each meal, and a little more during the meal. Then drink lots of water at night, as this will kill nighttime junk food cravings. Also, drink some water when you feel hungry to see if you were really thirsty.

Sleep Apnea: Starving for Sleep and Oxygen

There is a condition that many overweight people suffer from called sleep apnea. I personally had an extremely severe case of it; mine was almost life threatening. When you have sleep apnea, you stop breathing, sometimes hundreds of times, a night. You may not be aware that this is happening because you don't actually awaken, but it does disturb your sleep. The result is that you never get the full, rejuvenating benefits of a good night's sleep.

The reason that your breathing is interrupted is that the soft tissue in the rear of the throat collapses and cuts off the airway. This condition affects overweight people more because their neck is heavier, and the weight of the neck then collapses the airway. When I was at my heaviest, my neck measured twenty-two inches in diameter. No matter what position I lay in, once I started to fall asleep, I started suffocating. In the United States alone, millions of people have some degree of sleep apnea.[3]

Sleep apnea reduces blood oxygen to dangerously low levels, so your body is starving for oxygen. You become chronically exhausted, which causes junk food cravings. It also makes you more irritable and more prone to negative emotions that activate the FAT Programs. Just getting through the day when you have sleep apnea becomes a monumental challenge. I used to be so exhausted I would fall asleep in meetings, while driving my car, and while I was talking on the phone—even when I was the one talking!

Besides causing exhaustion and junk food cravings, sleep apnea elevates cortisol levels,[4] which activate the FAT Programs.[5] It is a vicious cycle; sleep apnea makes you fatter, and the fatter you get, the worse your sleep apnea becomes.

So what's the solution to sleep apnea and oxygen starvation?

Get Tested for Sleep Apnea

If you're in a position where you want to lose more than 100 pounds, chances are very strong that you have sleep apnea. Even if you're certain you don't have it because you think that you're sleeping well, please investigate the possibility in order to eliminate a potentially major stress on your body. If it turns out you have sleep apnea, having a sleep study test could easily be one of the most important nights of your life.

Sleep apnea is fully treatable, and if you have it, you MUST get it treated. In my opinion and experience, it is next to impossible to lose weight if you have untreated sleep apnea. The most common treatment is a CPAP machine, which is a machine that blows air into your nose and mouth while you sleep, keeping your airways unblocked. There are also other treatments that are similar.

The first step is to tell your doctor that you want to be tested for sleep apnea, and your doctor will refer you to a sleep study center. Typically, you'll spend a night in a hospital, where they'll monitor your sleeping and breathing patterns. The night of my sleep study test was one of the most memorable ones of my life. It was the first good night's sleep I had had in four or five years!

In most countries, both the sleep study and the CPAP machine are covered by insurance and/or Medicare.

Don't Eat Instead of Sleeping

Most people are tired in the late afternoons, when the FAT Programs are on, and this relates to low blood sugar episodes, which we'll talk more about in chapter 15. In addition to causing junk food cravings, low blood sugar can also cause exhaustion.

If at all possible, take a ten- or fifteen-minute catnap or listen to the Gabriel Method CD in the late afternoon. This can go a long way in solving your weight problems. You'll be less likely to eat junk food in the afternoon and late evening, you'll be less stressed out, and you'll be nourishing your body with the vital element of sleep.

Many people call these afternoon catnaps "power naps." I think this is a better way to refer to them because it takes the stigma out of sleeping in the afternoon. You are not being lazy; you are "power napping!" And you don't have to go home to have a power nap. Just get in your car, drive to a parking lot where no one knows you, lean back, and close your eyes and sleep or listen to the CD. Take a portable alarm clock with you, or program your cell phone to wake you up.

The later you stay up at night, the more likely it is you will start eating out of exhaustion. The best possible thing you can do for weight loss is to get to sleep before you reach that exhausted state.

NOTES

1. See D. Moore, "The Health Benefits of Drinking Water," Dr. Donnica Website (October 21, 2003): http://www.drdonnica.com/today/00007230.htm.

2. See K. Palma, "Got Water?" *The Eagle-Tribune* (April 24, 2002).

3. See Neal Friedman, Etta L. Fanning. *Disease Management.* September 1, 2004, 7 (supplement 1): S-1-S-6. doi:10.1089/dis.2004.7.S-1.

4. See http://www.battlediabetes.com/obstructive-sleep-apnea-linked-to-type-2-diabetes/.

5. See the appendix (page 185) for the relationship between cortisol and the FAT Programs.

14

Fat and Toxins

Your body uses fat to protect you from toxins. This is yet another example of the way that your body uses obesity to try to keep you safe.

A toxin is a non-nutritive and potentially harmful molecule, element, organism, or energy that your body must either eliminate or store in a safe place. Toxins come from our environment in the form of food, water, air, medications, electricity, and radiation. They are produced inside your body as a result of cellular mutations and also as a natural byproduct of your body's metabolic processes; these are just *natural* stresses. In the modern industrial world, the chemical assaults on our bodies are numerous indeed. According to one source:[1]

- some 77,000 chemicals are produced in North America alone;
- more than 3,000 chemicals are added to our food supply;
- more than 10,000 chemicals are used in the food processing industry; and
- one thousand new chemicals are introduced to the food industry each year.

These chemicals accidentally end up in our ground water, rivers, lakes, and oceans as well as deliberately in our food supply.

In some parts of the world, we are literally swimming in real poisons. Most of these chemicals and toxins are completely new, not only to our bodies but also to *nature*.

Our Stone Age bodies are not equipped to deal with Space Age poisons. Sometimes, in your body's attempt to neutralize poisons, it may inadvertently create new substances that are even more toxic than the original chemicals.

It's not your body's fault. It's doing the best it can to deal with things that don't even occur in nature.

There's a famous *I Love Lucy* episode where she and Ethel are working in the wrapping room in a chocolate factory. Of course, something goes wrong, and the conveyor belt that is bringing the chocolates to them starts going too fast for Lucy and Ethel to be able to wrap the candies. The humor comes from their increasingly desperate efforts to keep up with a system that's giving them more than they can handle. Lucy and Ethel end up stuffing bonbons in their mouths, into their uniforms, and into their hats, making their boss think they are doing a good job and inspiring him to speed up the conveyor belt even more.

Dealing with poisons in your body can be very similar. If you are living in a crowded city and eating a modern conventional diet, the toxins may be coming in much faster than your body can safely eliminate them. As a result, all these toxins have to be stored somewhere in the meantime. One of the places that your body stores toxins is in your fat cells because fat is a very effective chemical buffer. The fat surrounds the toxin and protects both the fat cell and the rest of your body from the potentially damaging effect of the toxin, until your body is ready to deal with the toxin.

One study found that most Americans are storing somewhere between four hundred and eight hundred toxic chemicals in their fat cells.[2]

Storing toxins in fat is supposed to be a temporary measure, a short-term solution. Your body is waiting for the day when it stops being overwhelmed by a toxic environment and has enough breathing space to get around to dealing with the toxic backlog. The problem is that if the toxic inflow just won't quit, tomorrow never comes, and the backlog keeps getting bigger and bigger.

Toxins can block your body's ability to burn fat, causing a resistance to losing weight. Another study reported that toxins can cause or exacerbate "insulin resistance,"[3] which is one of the mechanisms of your body's FAT Programs.[4]

Some of the greatest sources of toxins in our daily lives are the foods we eat. Modern, conventionally-farmed, processed foods are full of poisons, including pesticides, herbicides, binders, stabilizers, artificial flavor enhancers, and chemical fertilizers. They are also irradiated and genetically modified. Conventionally farmed, grain-fed meat is even worse due to all the toxins from the grains plus hormones, and it is chemically treated to look fresher longer. One of the tricks that meat packers are now using is the deadly poison carbon monoxide.[5] Carbon monoxide masks slime and decay, and also hides the smell of rotting meat.

What is more, not being able to digest food properly causes even more toxic overload as the foods decay in the intestines. Most modern foods cause excessive free radicals, which are other forms of toxins that need to be neutralized.

Toxins also cause inflammation. Some people believe that obesity is actually a "disease of inflammation"[6] because the hormones involved in inflammation also activate the FAT Programs.[7] Inflammation is a swelling of an area to protect an injury. When you think about it, obesity is often the exact same thing.

Medication

According to one doctor, the first lesson taught to medical students in pharmacology class is that all medicines are toxic to the body in some way.[8] The toxins in medicinal drugs can add to your toxic load, clog your liver, and make it that much harder for your body to burn fat.

While you must follow your doctor or healthcare professional's advice, I would urge you to have a conversation with your doctors to make sure they understand that you don't wish to overload your system with pills. You only want to take drugs *when absolutely necessary*. Always find out what natural alternatives are available. I'd also recommend that you be cautious about taking over-the-counter medications.

Cortisol Medication

Cortisol is one of the hormones that activates your FAT Programs. If you're taking any medication that either directly or indirectly increases the levels of the hormone cortisol in your body, that hormonal imbalance will undermine everything you're trying to achieve. Artificially increasing your cortisol levels for an extended period of time will activate the FAT Programs,[9] so, please ask your doctor if any medication you are taking can raise your cortisol levels.

Female Hormone Replacement Therapy (HRT)

HRT can also cause a resistance to weight loss. One woman told me that, for the last three months, she had gained weight, and she could not get her body to lose weight no matter what she did. I asked her if she was taking any female hormone replacement therapy, and it turned out that she just started taking progesterone about three months prior.

There are certainly pros and cons to female hormone replacement therapy, but the fact that it can cause a resistance to losing weight needs to be factored into the equation.

Food Additives

Artificial flavor enhancers like MSG are not only addictive,[10] causing you to eat more MSG-flavored food, but they activate the FAT Programs as well.[11] As a matter of fact, one of the ways researchers make a rat or mouse fat when they want to study obesity is to feed it MSG. There is even a term for it: MSG-induced obese rats.

MSG is in most seasoned, processed foods and is known by many different names, such as flavor enhancer 621, monosodium glutamate, and potassium glutamate. Additives that always contain MSG include hydrolyzed vegetable protein, hydrolyzed protein, hydrolyzed plant protein, plant protein extract, sodium caseinate, and calcium caseinate.[12]

Artificial Sweeteners

I recommend avoiding all artificial sweeteners. Saccharine (brand names such as Sweet'N Low and Sugarine) is carcinogenic.[13] Aspartame (brand name NutraSweet) is toxic to the brain,[14] can activate the FAT Programs,[15] is addictive, and also desensitizes the tongue to sugar so that it takes more sugar to make something taste sweet. Studies have even demonstrated that drinking diet soda with Aspartame can make you gain weight.[16] Sucralose (brand name Splenda) is made by adding chlorine to glucose, and many health experts are concerned about its use.[17]

I personally like the sweetener Xylitol. Xylitol is a natural sweetener usually derived from corncobs and birch bark. Xylitol really tastes like sugar, it has no bitter aftertaste, and you can cook with it. It does not cause blood sugar spikes like table sugar does, and it can actually help you lose weight. Xylitol helps turn off the FAT Programs by assisting the body in absorbing calcium[18] and by stabilizing insulin levels.[19] Because it assists the body in absorbing calcium, it can help improve teeth and bone density as well. Studies have actually shown that it can help reverse osteoporosis.[20]

Stevia is a natural, plant-based alternative sweetener, but frankly, I do not like the way it tastes. Raw honey is also a good natural alternative to table sugar but only if it is unprocessed. For my money, Xylitol is the sweetener of choice.

Vaccinations

The number and frequency of vaccinations most of us take has risen exponentially over the last twenty years at roughly the same rate as the obesity epidemic. While I cannot comment on the importance of every vaccination, one thing's for certain: they've got toxins in them. Most vaccinations contain formaldehyde, heavy metals, an untested cocktail of diseases incubated in monkey brains, and organ tissue surrogates derived from pigs and dogs. For me, a vaccination has to be a pretreatment for something that's absolutely life threatening before I will even consider it. Even then I would still rather rely on my body's natural defenses. Ultimately, you have to make a decision based on your doctor's advice and your own research, but please factor in the toxicity issue when you are deciding whether to get vaccinated or not.

Radiation

Our bodies use fat as a buffer to protect us against radiation as well. Once, when I was close to 400 pounds, I got a chest X-ray and the X-ray wasn't legible. The fat had absorbed the radiation before it could reach my organs. This is just another toxic, potential, FAT Programs activator.

What's the Solution for Toxicity?

We can reduce the inflow of toxins tremendously by eating more live, fresh, organic food. They have fewer toxins to begin with, and they are easier to digest. They also contain antioxidants that help neutralize free radicals. Water also helps flush out toxins. So following the approach outlined here will help you reduce the inflow of toxins and allow your body to start addressing the backlog that you have in your fat cells.

Eating more live foods will also help you detoxify because all live foods have fiber. This fiber will help clean out your colon and intestines of undigested food and stagnant waste.

NOTES

1. See J. Mercola and R. Droege, "How to Avoid the 10 Most Common Toxins," Mercola.com Newsletter (February 19, 2005): http://articles.mercola.com/sites/articles/archive/2005/02/19/common-toxins.aspx.

2. Ibid.

3. A. R. Ryalls, E. A. Berry, P. J. Manning, R. J. Walker, S. A. De Jong, S. M. Williams, and W. H. Sutherland, "Effect of High-Dose Vitamin E on Insulin Resistance and Associated Parameters in Overweight Subjects," *Diabetes Care* 27, no. 9 (American Diabetes Association, September 2004): 2166–2171.

4. See the appendix (page 185) for the relationship between insulin resistance and the FAT Programs.

5. See R. Weiss, "FDA is Urged to Ban Carbon-Monoxide-Treated Meat," *The Washington Post* (February 20, 2006).

6. See A. Ho, F. Nishimura, R. Genco, S. Grossi, and Y. Murayama: "A Proposed Model Linking Inflammation to Obesity, Diabetes, and Periodontal Infections," *Journal of Periodontology* 76, no. 11-s (American Academy of Periodontology, November 2005): 2075–2084; B. Wisse, "The Inflammatory Syndrome: The Role of Adipose Tissue Cytokine Metabolism in Metabolic Disorders Linked to Obesity," *Journal of the American Society of Nephrology* 15, no. 11 (2004): 2792–2800; and U. N. Das, "Is Obesity an Inflammatory Condition?" Nutrition 17, no. 11–12 (Elsevier, November–December 2001): 953–966.

7. See the appendix (page 185) for the relationship between proinflammatory cytokines and the FAT Programs.

8. See Joel Fuhrman, *Fasting and Eating for Health* (New York: St. Martin's Press, 1995).

9. See the appendix (page 185) for the relationship between chronically elevated cortisol levels and the FAT Programs.

10. See "MSG and Obesity," MSG Truth Website: http://www.msgtruth.org/obesity.htm.

11. Ibid.

12. See "What Foods to Avoid?" MSG Truth Website: http://www.msgtruth.org/avoid.htm.

13. See L. Shea, "Saccharin, Sweet'N Low and Cancer," BellaOnline Website (2008): http://www.bellaonline.com/articles/art15448.asp.

14. See B. Martini, "Beware of Ex[c]itotoxins: Diet Foods Can Ruin You," Pathlights Website (July 2002): http://www.pathlights.com/Public%20Enemies/other-nasties.htm.

15. Because aspartame is shaped chemically similar to sugar, it can trick the tongue into thinking it is sugar and cause an insulin response,

eventually leading to insulin resistance and hyperinsulinemia. Please see the appendix (page 185) for the relationship between hyperinsulinemia and the FAT Programs.

16. See "Diet Soda May Double Your Risk of Obesity," *San Antonio Express-News* (July 6, 2005).

17. See "The Potential Dangers of Sucralose," Mercola.com Newsletter (December 3, 2000): http://articles.mercola.com/sites/articles/archive/2000/12/03/sucralose-testimonials.aspx.

18. See M. M. Hämäläinen, "Bone Repair in Calcium-Deficient Rats: Comparison of Xylitol + Calcium Carbonate with Calcium Carbonate, Calcium Lactate and Calcium Citrate on the Repletion of Calcium," *The Journal of Nutrition* 124, no. 6 (American Society of Nutrition, June 1994): 874–881.

19. See H. Sato, M. Fujisawa, S. Katsuki, T. Asano, and Y. Hirata, "Effects of Intravenous Injection of Xylitol on Blood Sugar, Blood Pyruvic Acid and Plasma Insulin Levels in the Dog," *Research in Experimental Medicine* 145, no. 2 (Springer Berlin / Heidelberg, 1967): 111–119.

20. See D. Townsend, "Xylitol—Cavity-Fighting Sweetener Possible Solution for Osteoporosis," *Townsend Letter for Doctors and Patients* (May 1, 2002).

15

Easy Applications of the Principles in Part III

There is no one menu that is ideal for everyone. There is no correct amount of calories, and no correct proportion of carbohydrates, fats, and proteins that applies to all. Even focusing on calories, carbohydrates, fats, and proteins is a mistake because there are too many other issues that are more important.

For example, how much life force vitality does the food have? How uncorrupted are the nutrients? How digestible and assimilable are the nutrients for anyone in general and for you specifically? How does the way that you combine your food affect your ability to digest it? How many toxins are in your food? Does the food that you're eating have a detoxifying effect on your body, or does it increase your body's toxic load? How does the food you are eating alter the level of the FAT Program hormones,[1] and how does it affect your body's sensitivity to these hormones?

How fast are you eating your food? What time of day are you eating your food? How frequently are you eating? How conscious are you when you are eating? Are you consciously and thoroughly chewing your food, or are you mindlessly putting it into your mouth while watching TV?

These are all questions that need to be factored into the equation. I don't mean to make it sound too complicated, because the solutions are simple. But the solutions do not lie in counting calories, carbohydrates, fats, and proteins, which is what all diets do, and they usually stop right there.

Applying the Principles Is Not Hard

As a general rule, a good meal should have three ingredients in it—protein, omega-3 fatty acids, and live food. If you have these three elements, you will be more nourished, less toxic, less hungry, and you will eliminate many of the physical stresses and starvation signals that activate your FAT Programs. Anytime you are eating a meal, ask yourself three questions:

1. Where's the protein?
2. Where's the live food?
3. Where are the omega-3s?

The presence of these three factors does something else that is crucial for weight loss: they keep your blood sugar levels stable for long periods of time. When your FAT Programs are on, you lose the ability to regulate your blood sugar properly. This is because the cells of your body become resistant to the hormone insulin, so your insulin levels start to rise. Insulin is the fat storage hormone, and it prevents your body from burning fat efficiently. Everybody's so focused on calories in and calories out, no one even bothers to ask the question "Do I even have the ability to burn fat at all?" And when your insulin levels are too high, the answer is no, not really.

You also lose the ability to keep your blood sugar levels stable when your insulin levels are too high. Elevated insulin levels cause frequent low blood sugar episodes that lead to exhaustion and ravenous junk food cravings (just think about how you sometimes feel at three or four in the afternoon, or late at night). "Dead carbs" cause your blood sugar levels to spike, and this makes your insulin levels rise even higher only to cause your blood sugar to plummet an hour or two later. The result: further carb cravings. That's why you're sometimes hungry for sweets a little while after eating a big meal with lots of dead carbs. You end up eating again, not because you need more calories, but simply because you can't keep your blood sugar levels up.

Protein, live food, and omega-3s keep your blood sugar levels stable for long periods of time, so you don't get wild blood sugar fluctuations and unnecessary sugar cravings. They also help your body start to become more sensitive to insulin, and this causes your insulin levels to come back down to normal.

Lots of great things happen when your insulin levels normalize. You regain the ability to burn fat efficiently AND you maintain the ability to keep your blood sugar levels stable. As a result, you have more energy and fewer junk food cravings, and you start living off of your fat reserves instead of having to make the junk food industry endlessly richer. It's a win/win scenario.

So always ask yourself in every meal: Where's the protein, where's the live food, and where are the omega-3s? Remember that the focus is always on adding. Adding, adding, adding. Even if you're eating junk and especially if your eating dead carbs, add foods that have these things, and they will help prevent the blood sugar peaks and troughs.

In addition to including live foods, protein, and omega-3s, I would also try to incorporate the other eating and drinking suggestions found at the end of each chapter in this section, such as taking omega-3 capsules, probiotics, and digestive enzymes. Fermented foods are also typically very good for you, such as miso, tempeh, tamari, and brewer's yeast. And don't forget to drink plenty of pure water—preferably natural, nongaseous spring water.

Super Delicious, Super Nutritious

On my website you'll find lots of Super Nutritious, Super Delicious recipes. The idea is that I can take virtually any recipe, replace dead/toxic ingredients with superhealthy ingredients, and make it taste just as good—if not better—than the original. Just go to gabrielmethod.com/recipes.

Listen to Your Body's Signals

If you learn to listen to your body's signals, it will tell you if the food you are eating is nourishing you or causing hormonal chaos. Pay very close attention to how you feel an hour after a meal. Do you feel energized and satisfied, or do you feel exhausted and hungry? Did the food hit the spot or was it just a short-term fix? How do you feel emotionally? Are you in a good mood, or are you irritable and cranky?

These signs will tell you whether the foods you are eating are nourishing you; they will tell you if you are eating the right fuel.

Shift Your Hunger Habit

Our bodies are designed to use the food we eat during the day as energy for that day. What we don't use during the day, we have to store. This means that we are actually supposed to eat our food during the day and not at night, when it is time to sleep.

However, when the FAT Programs are on, certain hormones that are supposed to decline in the evenings become elevated instead. This causes excessive nighttime hunger and junk food cravings.[2] It is highly likely the body causes this hormonal disturbance deliberately when the FAT Programs are on *because eating at night is the best way to make you fat!*

Also, when you eat excessively at night, your insulin levels stay elevated while you sleep. Insulin is the fat storage hormone, so your body stays in fat storage mode all night. In essence, you end up making fat while you sleep.

If your stomach is not full when you go to sleep, your body will be burning fat at night. So the difference between eating your food at night and eating it during the day is the difference between making fat all night and burning it all night. You can eat the same foods and the same amount, but if you just eat earlier, you can potentially lose weight on the same amount of food.

When you turn off the FAT Programs, you will no longer have the hormonal problems that cause excessive nighttime hunger. But you may still be in the habit of eating at night. You can easily shift your hunger habit by eating larger meals during the day. After a few days, your body will fall into the habit of being hungrier in the morning and afternoon, and less so at night. It will come to expect that the majority of the food you eat is eaten during the day, and because it expects the main meal to be in the morning or afternoon, it actually gets hungrier at those times.

The way to start changing your hunger habits is to make an effort to eat a large breakfast with lots of protein, live food, and omega-3s. In doing so, you will have gotten all of the essential nutrients that you need in an uncorrupted and highly digestible form. Therefore, first thing in the morning, you have already given your body everything it needs. This means you will no longer be perpetually starving for nutrients.

Have lots of "real" food snacks in the afternoons. Over time, as you find that you are getting hungrier in the mornings and afternoons, and less so at night, make it a point to eat smaller, lighter, healthier, and earlier dinners. The key is to eat a lot of food during the day and to drink a lot of water at night, which will help banish hunger pangs.

After dinner, drink a glass of water every hour or so. In this way, you'll start shifting your hunger habits. Then you'll be eating all you want and as much as you want, and you'll be losing weight instead of gaining.

Conscious Eating

When the FAT Programs are on, your body reacts as if it's a time of famine. This causes you to eat each meal as if you may not see food again for days or weeks. That's why fat people often eat so fast and furiously. I can tell you that I have never seen anyone eats as quickly and as ferociously as I used to eat when my body wanted to be fat. I ate each meal as if I had not seen food in a month. When you eat leisurely, you are sending a message to your body that "food is abundant, it is not a time of famine, and there is no need to hurry or overeat."

Also, it takes about twenty minutes for your brain to get the message your stomach is full. In those twenty minutes, you can pack into your stomach twice as much food as you would otherwise want or need, and what happens next is that you stretch your stomach. When you stretch your stomach, it takes even more food to fill it. You end up having to eat more food just to feel full, but this feeling has nothing to do with how much food you actually need.

The way to avoid these problems is to eat leisurely and more consciously. Rather than mechanically putting food into your mouth while you are watching TV or reading, become aware of the fact that you are actually eating.

Make a real effort to chew your food thoroughly and really taste it—see if you can identify each spice used. I find that cooking with new and unfamiliar spices is a good way to train the taste buds to turn back on. When you chew your food more thoroughly, you digest it much better. Digestion begins in your mouth. There are digestive enzymes in the saliva that will help predigest the food you're eating. By digesting your food better, you'll be extracting more nutrients out of the food, and you will, therefore, require less food to nourish yourself.

If you think about it, this should not really be a chore, because all of the fun of eating is when the food is actually in your mouth, and you actually taste it. By keeping the food in your mouth longer, you're maximizing the pleasure of the meal.

Additionally, after eating for about five or ten minutes, it's a good idea to take a short break. Just relax, and enjoy your surroundings or the company you are with. This reinforces the message to your body that food is abundant; there is no need to rush. It also gives your brain a chance to catch up with your stomach.

Lettuce Slow You Down

One great strategy for making your meals more abundant is to turn them into salads. Leafy greens take a long time to chew, so you can't help but chew your food more thoroughly and more slowly when it's in the form of a salad.

For example, if you are eating a pizza, you can cut the pizza up into bite-sized chunks and put them into a salad with lots of different fresh lettuce leaves and sprouts. Choose a dressing that you really love and use as much as you want. Remember, we're not counting calories; we're trying to develop the habit of eating more slowly. As an added bonus, you'll develop the habit of eating and loving salads. This way, you're eating more slowly, you're eating less, you're eating healthier, you're digesting your food better, and you're still enjoying it just as much.

You can turn almost anything into a salad if you want, even fast food! All you have to do is cut it up and put it in a bowl, adding lots of healthy leafy greens, maybe some sprouts, and a delicious dressing. I recommend using flaxseed oil (or another nut or seed oil) in your dressing; you can also add protein powder to any creamy dressing to increase the nutritional content of your meal.

Whether you adopt the salad strategy or not, please make a conscious effort to eat more leisurely and to chew your food thoroughly.

Eat Like a Thin Person

So-called "naturally thin" people eat what they want, whenever they want, and they don't beat themselves over the head because of it.

I suggest that you eat what you want without judgment, hesitation, or guilt. By doing this, you de-emphasize the relationship that you have with food. De-emphasize the relationship, and you'll weaken the control food has on you. In this way, you'll eliminate binging, and you'll have no "good days" and no "bad days." Eventually the whole issue will go away, and you'll be a naturally thin person.

Have a Ten-Minute Super-Vitality Break

One final suggestion for tying together the information in this section is that you try to have a ten-minute Super-Vitality Break every day or as often as possible. Maybe try after lunch, or in the afternoon, when your energy is lagging, or in the late morning after you have done some work.

In that ten-minute break, go to a juice bar and have a shot of fresh wheatgrass juice, which is full of live chlorophyll. Live chlorophyll is pure liquid vitality. It's basically energy from the sun that's converted into essential nutrients. It's like drinking captured sunlight—most likely the best thing you can put in your body. If you don't like the taste of wheatgrass juice, you can mix it in a glass of water, or in vegetable or fruit juice, and you will not even know that it's there.

You can also grow wheatgrass, or buy it by the tray and juice it yourself. That's what I do. I have a wheatgrass juicer, and I buy a set number of trays every week. For maximum effect, the wheatgrass has to be freshly squeezed and drunk within two minutes of being squeezed; otherwise, you lose all the enormous benefits of the vitality. I'm always amazed at how different the juice tastes if I wait more than two minutes to drink it; it loses all of its taste. But juice that's freshly squeezed and drunk right away is quite nice. Another important point to consider when buying wheatgrass juice is that some juice bars precut the grass, keep it in the refrigerator, and then juice it. While this might be more convenient for them, it's less preferable in terms of both taste and benefits.

If, for whatever reason, it is not possible for you to get wheatgrass juice, have some live, fresh, dark greens.

That's one part of the equation for the Super-Vitality Break. The other part is to go outside for five minutes and practice the Chi-Kung technique "Eating the Sun" that I described in chapter 11. Just that ten-minute exercise will boost your energy so that you are not exhausted in the afternoons and evenings. As a result, you will no longer have the energy lulls that cause junk food cravings. In addition, you'll be super-charging your body with the essential life force energy we all need.

These simple suggestions will enable you to eliminate the physical forms of starvation and toxic overload that can make your body want to be fat, and that turn on the FAT Programs. As your body gets more nourished, it gets healthier and strays away from the need to be fat. You'll notice that you'll gradually become less hungry, you'll crave healthier foods, you'll have more energy, and you'll be naturally more active and interested in living a more physical lifestyle.

Your body will also start to burn fat more and more efficiently. A positive spiral develops because, the better your body gets at burning fat, the more energy you will have and the less food you'll need. Whenever your body needs some energy, it can just tap into your fat reserves, rather than force you to get it from outside sources.

As these things come together, you'll be losing weight without even having to make an effort to be disciplined or "in control" of yourself. Your body will be working with you, as opposed to against you, in your weight-loss effort.

In the final section of this book, we'll talk about how to phase these suggestions into your life and make them into habits. Before you know it, they will become an automatic part of your daily life.

NOTES

1. See the appendix (page 185) for the relevant hormones involved in the FAT Programs.

2. For more on how the binaural rhythm of cortisol levels gets reversed so that cortisol levels stay elevated at night, see S. Talbott, *The Cortisol Connection* (Alameda, CA: Hunter House Publishers, 2002); and the appendix (page 185) for the relationship between cortisol and the FAT Programs.

PART IV

Positive Forces That Make Your Body *Want* to Be Thin

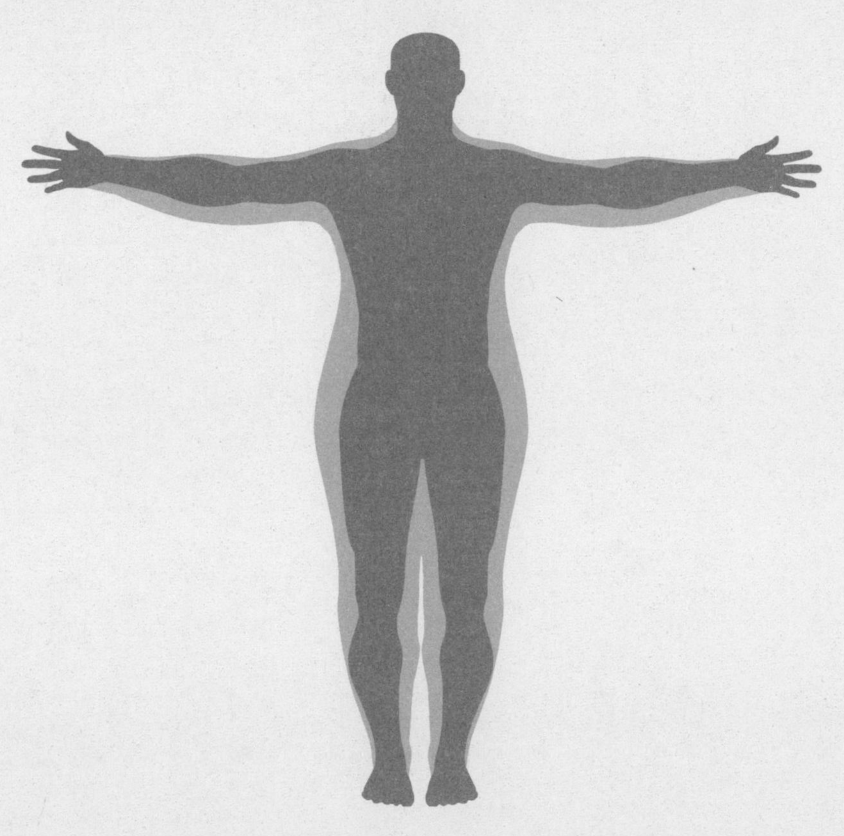

16

The Positive Stresses

Up until now, we have been focusing our attention on how to eliminate the negative stresses (both physical and emotional) that can activate the FAT Programs. These are the stresses that trick your body into thinking it needs to be fat in order to protect you. But just as your body can be tricked into thinking it needs to be fat, it can just as easily be tricked into thinking, "I need to be thin!"

As far as weight loss is concerned, stress can be a good thing or a bad thing. That's why stress will make some people fatter and other people thinner. With mental and emotional stresses, it often depends on the way your brain interprets those stresses. However, there are some stresses where the interpretation can really only go one way: "we need to be thinner in order to survive." Or to put it more fundamentally: Get thin or get eaten.

Get Thin or Get Eaten

When you introduce stresses that cause your body to believe it has to be thin in order to survive, you've won the weight-loss battle. These are the good stresses. And there are ways you can make these stresses a welcome part of your daily life.

Let's first look at the principle stress that will make your body want to be thin: exercise.

WARNING LETTER

Dear Reader,

Hi! It's me, your friendly author.

I know.

I've used the "E" word.

Right now, you may hate exercise. Most people do. Believe me, I once hated it just as much as you do, and I know what you're thinking:

"OH (insert your favorite four-letter word)!!!!!!"

"Up until now everything was going great!"

"I KNEW THERE WAS A CATCH!!!!!!!!!!!"

But please hear me out. I am not going to ask you to exercise if you don't want to. I only want to point out some interesting facts that you may not be aware of regarding exercise.

I also have some useful pointers for you on how to get the biggest bang for your buck from exercise, as well as how to get the most fun out of it. So if you choose to exercise, you will get very quick results. You will also begin to enjoy exercise rather than dread it.

When I weighed over 400 pounds, I'd practically pass out trying to tie my shoelaces. Not only was moving not fun but breathing was even hard. Exercise was the last thing on my mind—right behind trying "The Arctic Jellyfish Diet."

But you have to understand. Besides the obvious and strictly mechanical challenges that make moving difficult and so unpleasant when you're overweight, there are also very definite chemical and psychological factors at work here—factors that can cause you to hate exercise.

For one thing, when the FAT Programs are on, your body doesn't want you to exercise because exercising will help you lose weight. And that's the last thing that your body wants you to do.

Remember, one of the chief components of the FAT Programs is to force you to conserve energy. Your body makes you feel tired all the time. This is a deliberate mechanism your body uses to keep you inactive. When the FAT Programs are on, just even thinking about exercise will make you feel tired.

We have talked at length about the many ways you can turn off the FAT Programs, so once these issues have been resolved, the chemical and hormonal component of the "I hate exercise" equation will naturally go away. You will have much more energy, you will experience a new spring in your step, and you will actually want to exercise and be more active; that takes care of the chemical component.

But there's still the psychological component. There are still a whole host of negative associations you may have related to exercise. You also have to address those associations before you can really enjoy exercise.

So bear with me, and hang in there for a little while longer.

Yours truly,
Jon

Exercise—The Best Stress of All to Make Your Body Want to Be Thin

Exercise is valuable not because it burns calories but because, if done correctly, it can actually make your body want to be thin.

Everyone knows exercise burns calories, but simply burning calories is useless if all it does is make you hungrier. If you burn more calories but you also need to eat more food, the net effect is zero.

From a weight-loss perspective, the calories you burn during exercise are only a *very minor consideration* compared with the many other positive benefits exercise provides. In fact, focusing on the calorie burning aspect of exercise can be discouraging and demoralizing. At the gym, there's an aerobic machine that's supposed to be able to tell me how many calories I've burned, but whenever I use it I feel discouraged. I'm amazed at how few calories I've burned compared to the amount of effort I've put in.

In reality, the machine can't possibly calculate how many calories I've burned during the workout since it knows nothing about what's happening at a biochemical level inside my body. The machine is only measuring calories in terms of the mechanical work I'm doing, which is based on a calculation of my age and body weight. This number is truly meaningless. A body with twice as much muscle might burn twice as many calories—or more—doing the same exercise. Even if the measure were more accurate, it would be no indication of how much fat you are burning.

A body that's resistant to using its fat reserves as fuel will burn much less fat per calories used than a highly-trained, athletic body. If you pay attention to this counterproductive gimmick, you'll be left with the feeling it's better to just eat three hundred calories less in a day than to exercise for an hour. And as you should know by now, nothing could be further from the truth!

The calories burned during a workout are not relevant. Just like our food's hormonal effects are more important to consider than the calories of what we eat, the hormonal effects of exercise are more important than the calories we burn during exercise.[1]

How the Right Exercise Makes Your Body Want to Be Thin

Your body wants to be thin when it thinks that it must be thin in order to survive. If you were living in an environment where there were man-eating animals chasing you and every couple of days or so you had to make a run for it to escape being eaten, your body would understand that you need to be thin and fast, and that the thinner you are the safer you will be. Even having *1 ounce* of excess fat could be the difference between life and death. The right exercise can ambush your body into thinking that you are living in such an environment. It will make your body think it must be as thin and as fit as possible in order to survive.

When you're playing a sport and you run as fast as you can to try to get the ball, your body assumes you're doing so for only one reason: survival. Imagine for a moment that you're playing soccer, and you get the ball thirty meters from the goal. You sprint with all your might to outrun the defender, and you take the shot—Score!!! What you've just done, in that instance, is cause the exact same hormonal signals in your body that mimic running away from a lion in the African savannah.

Your body has no idea that you're voluntarily sprinting because you're trying to score a goal. It doesn't know what a game of soccer is or what a goal is, and it doesn't care. If you're moving that quickly and with such intense urgency, the only conclusion your body can make is that you must be doing so in order to stay alive. If you need to put on these sudden bursts of speed, your body will conclude that you are living in a place where there are predators lurking about.

The Right Exercise to Deactivate the FAT Programs

You can take advantage of this survival response and exploit it as a tool to make your body want to be thin.

The right exercise isn't simply a calorie-burning device; the right type of exercise turns off the FAT Programs. And here's some good news: you don't have to exercise excessively.

Don't exercise longer; just exercise smarter!

Health Departments in the United States now recommend doing light aerobics for an hour a day, six or seven days a week. They are making this recommendation because they only see exercise as a calorie-burning tool. Now, light aerobics are great, but imagine you were walking along in the forest and a bear came out of nowhere. Would you go for a forty-minute, light aerobic walk? No, you'd move as fast as you could for a few seconds or a few minutes until you had either outrun the bear or your friends, who the bear is also chasing. In the same way, whenever you're being physically active, it's those very brief moments of intensity that make your body think that you need to be thin.

Leisurely walking is great because it *does* burn calories, increases blood circulation and cardio fitness, and it strengthens your muscles. I recommend it and I do not mean to belittle it; it's very useful. But it will not necessarily make your body want to be thin. And that is our primary objective—to make your body want to be thin.

Walking can be a great exercise. But when you're going for a walk, the way to maximize the benefit of the walk is to vary the speed at which you are walking periodically. So if you're going for a twenty-minute walk, don't just push yourself straight through for the whole twenty minutes. It's much better to go at a leisurely pace for the majority of the time and then three or four times during the walk, walk a little faster for thirty seconds or a minute. It is in those brief periods when you are moving faster that you are able to make your body think that its survival is at risk. As far as your body is concerned, the hormonal message is loud and clear:

Alert! Alert! Nothing is more important than being lean and fast! The predators chasing us could kill us at any moment! Forget about storing and holding onto fat! We have new priorities! Drop weight! Do whatever you can to drop weight! Shut off all the FAT Programs, and get thin NOW!!

One recent study monitored women who exercised on a stationary bike for twenty minutes a day, three times a week. The women were told to sprint for eight to twelve seconds periodically during their ride. Interestingly, these women lost three times as much weight as women who exercised at a continuous pace for forty minutes.[2]

Visualization Techniques for Maximizing the Weight-loss Benefits of Exercise

If you really want to get the most out of exercise in the briefest amount of time, do this:

The Imaginary Predator

One day I went out for a bike ride and I was feeling kind of flat. My ride was boringly routine, and I thought that I needed something to pick it up and keep me motivated. No sooner did I have that thought when a dog came running out of its driveway and started chasing me. I immediately stood up and began sprinting as fast as I could. The dog stayed with me for almost a mile, sometimes just inches away from taking a bite out my Achilles tendon. He eventually gave up, and the rest of my ride was phenomenal. I had gotten all the motivation and excitement I needed, and I was really pumped up.

Over the next few weeks, I noticed that my fitness had made a quantum leap. I was much stronger, and my typical ride was easy as could be. It then occurred to me that I had just connected with something very primal. For those brief few moments, my body was running for its life, and so it adapted by getting leaner and stronger. After this event, I started doing something different. Every time I got to that point in my ride, I would stand up and imagine that the dog was chasing me. I discovered that this is a great way to activate the get thin or get eaten adaptation response. For me, the dog chase gave me the same benefits as a similar experience had given to Jessie, my cat.

Technique: So in those brief moments during exercise when you're moving at your fastest, imagine that a predator is actually chasing you and you're moving so fast because you're running for your life.

Your body doesn't know the difference between real and imagined threats, so it won't know you are making up this visualization in your head. It will think that something *is* really chasing you and that your life is at stake. Being thin and fast is now a matter of life and death. As a result, you'll get much more out of your workout than simply burning a few calories. And exercise already puts you in SMART Mode, so visualizations during exercise are very effective.

Your Ideal Body

Technique: Whenever you're physically active, you can visualize your ideal body. Usually at some point while biking, I will imagine that I am in my ideal shape. I imagine that I can see every stomach muscle, and that the veins and muscles in my arms are bulging. Use whatever image of your ideal self that works for you.

Alternating between these two visualization techniques during the times when you are moving faster will help maximize the benefits of your exercise session. It will make your body think it needs to be thin in order to survive, and it will program your body to be in perfect shape.

Nighttime Visualization to Rekindle the Joy of Movement

All children love to play. At a certain age, we just love being physically active. But even if we lose that joy, the good news is that we can find it again.

Technique: At night, before you go to sleep or whenever you're in SMART Mode, do this:

- Imagine you are in perfect shape and you already have your ideal body.
- Imagine that you have no physical limitations. Being active is as effortless and as enjoyable as when you were a small child.
- Choose a physical activity that really appeals to you; it can be anything at all. Maybe it's something you've

always dreamed of doing, such as skiing, surfing, hang gliding, skydiving, or mountain climbing. You can even win gold medals at the Olympics in swimming, sprinting, pole vaulting, or gymnastics—whatever you want.

- Whatever you're visualizing, use all your senses. Feel the wind, taste the water, smell the fresh-cut grass, hear the sound of the turns you make on the snow—feel every part of your body alive with the joy of movement.

Overtraining—Don't Exercise Too Much!

If you exercise too frequently and/or too long, exercise becomes a negative stress that can actually activate the FAT Programs.

Overdoing exercise is called overtraining, and its effects are well documented. Many studies have shown that athletes will continue to get in better shape from exercise until they start exercising too much.[3] When that happens, they actually begin *gaining* weight. The reason is that overtraining elevates cortisol[4] levels, and cortisol turns on the FAT Programs.[5]

The most glaring example of overtraining I've ever seen came from my friend Sasha. A year after Sasha had given birth, she still had an extra 30 pounds that she could not shed. Sasha became an exercise maniac, doing two, one-hour exercise videos a day, six days a week. After a few months of grinding away for hours a day, day after day, she really started to resent it. Yet, because of her tremendous endurance and perseverance, she kept going and going, like paying a toll each day just for existing.

Because Sasha exercised too long and too often, she became overtrained and wasn't losing any more weight. Eventually, she hit the wall. She just couldn't go on beating herself up every day, and she was forced to let the whole thing go. Over the next three months, Sasha lost those thirty pounds without doing one stitch of exercise. It just fell off her.

When she removed the chronic mental and physical stress of a punishing exercise routine from her life, Sasha allowed her body to return to its naturally thin state. This is a really important point for all those "no pain, no gain" and "more is better" people out there:

Just like *forcing* yourself to diet will backfire, *forcing* yourself to exercise can have the same detrimental results and for exactly the same reasons.

So, when it comes to exercise, it's not always about more, more, more. You need rest days. Your body will then be fresh and enthusiastic so you will no longer dread being physically active. The idea is to learn to love exercising again. If you embrace the joy of being physical again, it no longer becomes a chore, and it will then stay with you for life.

If you do decide to exercise, don't overdo it! Make sure you rest at least three days a week. I personally like biking. I have a beautiful ride I do through the local vineyards. I usually do the ride three days a week. Sometimes I take a yoga class Saturday mornings. The other days of the week, I rest and let my body regenerate, so I am always fresh and enthusiastic about my rides. If I ever lose that enthusiasm, I take off a few days or a week to relax. Now, I sometimes go weeks at a time without exercising, but I always come back to it because I now truly love being physically active. I love the way my body feels when I am doing it and afterwards. I just feel happier, and life just becomes easier.

Tips for Getting Started

If you decide you would like to start living a more physically active life, here are three good tips:

- **Be open to the possibility that your body is changing.** When your body no longer wants to be fat, you'll have more energy and enthusiasm, and you'll want to be active. This could happen at any time along the path. It could happen immediately, after listening to the CD just once, or it could happen in six months time. You just have to be open to the possibility that this shift in your feelings about exercise is imminent. Stay open to the idea, and always keep an eye out for some type of activity that would be fun. When you find such an activity, give yourself the opportunity to experience fun and to reconnect with your body.

- **Visualize.** The night before exercising, visualize the next day by seeing yourself enjoying the activity of choice. If you are going to play basketball, see yourself putting on your outfit, tying your shoes, going to the court, and having a great time. See yourself in great shape as you are playing. Take advantage whenever you can to do the other visualizations as well—the Imaginary Predator, Your Ideal Body, and Rekindling the Joy.
- **Have an inspirational role model.** For me, as I was losing weight, that inspiration was Ashrita Furhman. Ashrita has broken over 186 world records for feats involving superhuman strength and endurance. He holds the world record for the fastest time running fifty miles while juggling! He pole-vaulted up Mount Fuji. He holds the record for the fastest mile while balancing a milk bottle on his head. The list goes on and on. He once biked for over twenty-four hours straight after training only three days!

  When I first read about Ashrita, I was spellbound that it was humanly possible to do such things. He was, and still is, a tremendous inspiration for me. I remember when I first started biking, I would think to myself: if Ashrita can bike for twenty-four hours, then certainly I can bike for twenty minutes. This put everything in perspective for me and made it all much easier.

Finally, always get your doctor's approval before starting an exercise program.

Other Ways to Maximize the "Get Thin or Get Eaten" Adaptation

Aside from the right type of exercise, there is another way to connect with that primal "Get thin!" adaptation. You can trigger an "acute stress." An acute stress is any sudden and intense stress, and it can be frightening, exciting, or thrilling.

The very first acute stress was the stress of running away from a predator—the "fight or flight" response. Studies show that periodic acute stresses turn off the FAT Programs.[6]

Become an Adrenaline Junkie

One of the best-known phenomena associated with fight or flight is the adrenaline rush—that feeling of excited euphoria that makes you feel, "Whoa! I'm glad I survived that!"

Thrill seekers are "adrenalin junkies," or people who are hooked on the feeling of an adrenaline rush. Have you ever noticed that thrill seekers are usually thin? This is because thrills are acute stresses that cause the same kind of adrenalin surge that we would get if a lion were chasing us.

Activities like bungee jumping or parachuting cause the same kind of heart-pounding, emergency response. Our bodies assume that a predator is chasing us, that we must be living in an environment where danger is lurking, and therefore, we must be thin in order to survive.

Of course, these are extreme examples, but anything that excites you or makes you feel alive can be useful for creating that ideal stress. Other good examples include balloon rides, ferris wheels, roller-coaster rides, and paint ball. Taking a cold shower works too. Events that make you feel a little nervous will also do the trick, like giving a presentation. You may be nervous at first and during your speech, but afterwards you may feel relieved, or even exhilarated and euphoric.

A perfect example of how thrill seeking can make your body want to be thin is Jack Osbourne, son of famed rocker Ozzie Osbourne and star of the reality TV show *The Osbournes*. Jack fell in love with rock climbing and lost fifty-five pounds in just a few months time. His immediate transformation clearly demonstrates the effectiveness of thrill seeking for connecting to that primal instinct that makes your body want to be thin.

Get Your Brain to Interpret Stress the Right Way

Use the everyday stresses of your life to your advantage; you can turn a bad stress into a good stress. The next time you're at the office and you find out that the stock market crashed, or that the client from hell is screaming down the phone and blaming you for all his personal problems, take the first available opportunity to do something physical right then and there, on the spot. Two minutes is all it takes. Walk up a few flights of stairs, or go outside and move—react physically. What you're doing is telling your body that the stress you've just experienced was a predator you had to run away from.

Remember, it's not the mental threat or the fear that matters; it's the way that our animal brains interpret the threat. Is it something you have to run away from quickly, or is it something chronic and ongoing that will make your body think that perhaps being fatter will help keep you safe? When you react by moving your body, your animal brain is more likely to think, "We don't know what the threat is, but she's moving. She's not just sitting there taking it. It must be an attack. This has been happening a lot lately, so we'd better start to get thin!"

So when you experience a sudden stress, react to it immediately. With two minutes of physical movement you will be turning a negative stress—a stress that could otherwise make your body want to be fatter—into a positive stress, one that will make your body want to be thinner.

NOTES

1. See C. Yamamoto, K. Yamanouchi, N. Sakamoto, S. Hayamizu, Y. Ohkuwa, and Y. Sato, "Improved Insulin Sensitivity in Carbohydrate and Lipid Metabolism After Physical Training," *International Journal of Sports Medicine*, 7, no. 6 (Thieme, December 1986): 307–310. For more on how exercise lowers triglycerides, see L. Kravitz and V. Heyward, "The Exercise & Cholesterol Controversy," *IDEA Today* 12, no. 2 (IDEA Health & Fitness Association, 1994): 38–42; W. L. Haskell, "The Influence of Exercise on the Concentrations of Triglyceride and Cholesterol in Human Plasma," *Exercise and Sport Sciences Reviews*, 12 (Lippincott, Williams & Wilkins, 1984): 205–244. To read a more in-depth discussion about how exercise helps relieve stress and improve cortisol metabolism, see S. Talbott, *The Cortisol Connection* (Alameda, CA:

Hunter House Publishers, 2002): 44–45; and the appendix (page 185) for the relationship between insulin resistance, triglycerides, cortisol, and the FAT Programs.

2. See D. J. Chisholm, E. G. Trapp, J. Freund, and S. H. Boutcher, "The Effects of High-Intensity Intermittent Exercise Training and Fat Loss and Fasting Insulin Levels of Young Women," *International Journal of Obesity* 32 (Nature Publishing Group, January 15, 2008): 684–691.

3. See E. R. Eichner, "Overtraining: Consequences and Prevention," *Journal of Sports Science*, 13, no. 1, supp. 1 (Routledge, Summer 1995): s41–s48.

4. See note 1 above: S. Talbott.

5. See the appendix (page 185) for the relationship between elevated cortisol levels and the FAT Programs.

6. See B. Youngblood, D. Ryan, J. Simpson, R. Harris, S. Redmann, Jr., and T. Mitchell, "Weight Loss in Rats Exposed to Repeated Acute Restraint Stress is Independent of Energy or Leptin Status," *American Journal of Physiology—Regulatory, Integrative, and Comparative Physiology* 282, no. 1 (American Physiological Society, January 2002): R77–R88.

17

Success Profiles: The Gabriel Method in Practice

The Gabriel Method was first published in Australia in February 2007. Since that time, I've been flooded with stories from people who have lost weight and totally transformed their bodies and their lives. I've chosen a small sample of men and women in various age groups who demonstrate the types of results that you can expect to achieve. Some of them lost weight very quickly, some gradually, but all of them have learned that their weight problems were never really about discipline or calorie control. It was always about some other aspect of their lives that needed to be addressed. Many of them I've had personal contact with, and I've included them because they are so near and dear to my heart.

Carol Skabe is my daughter's nanny. She was the first person (besides me) to use the Gabriel Method, and I consider her to be one of my guardian angels. I remember when Carol came into my life. It was at a time when I was spending twelve to fifteen hours a day writing and doing biochemistry research on the internet, and I was unable to give my daughter all the time and attention she needed. Carol came out of nowhere and gave my daughter so much more than time. Carol gave my daughter her presence and validation.

They were together nearly every day, and their love for each other went far beyond that of a child and her caretaker. She also offered Inge an extended family of two aunts and seven grandchildren, all of them loving her and fighting for her attention. There are no words to describe how grateful I am that Carol is in my life. I'm so happy I was able to give something back to her. Here is her story.

I Deserve the Best for Myself

I was battling with my weight problems, probably from the age of ten—fluctuating all the time.

Being a girl, I wanted to wear the sort of clothes other girls were wearing, but I couldn't. So when I became a teenager, I felt unattractive and inadequate. And because of having weight problems for most of my life, I didn't feel good enough. I didn't feel good about myself or about the way I felt when I looked at myself. And in the long run, I think that I made some mistakes with my relationships. I didn't feel adequate enough, therefore I wasn't attracting the best men into my life. And I didn't feel that I deserved better.

I tried all sorts of weight-loss programs and I always did lose weight in the beginning, but then I always put it back on. I tried calorie counting and all the other ways of doing things, short of starving myself, and I had sugar cravings all the time.

Eventually, I just needed to try something different. Jon's method seemed pretty basic because it wasn't a diet; it just focused on eating properly. I wasn't feeling healthy at all. I wasn't energetic enough. I needed to feel better physically and better about myself emotionally. I needed peace of mind. So I gave it a go.

I started eating what Jon calls "real food" and thought at the beginning, "Well, this apple could not possibly compensate for a bar of chocolate, and this is a lot of rubbish because I'm still hungry." But after about a week, I found that I wanted the fruit and that it tasted better than chocolate. He also told me to sprinkle ground flaxseeds on everything, which I didn't mind at all. And with the help of Jon's visualization CD, I started waking up in the morning feeling better, more positive about myself. I found it wasn't only a weight-loss CD but it was also a positive affirmation. I was more positive about the food that I was eating and about the way my day was going. I'd get more done in a day, my energy level was going up, and the weight was coming off; I could see it coming off me. And if I did falter a little bit, it wasn't bad, because, with all the good food that I was eating, my body was still getting the nutrition it needed.

One thing that Jon taught me was not to feel guilty, but I was craving junk food less and less anyhow.

I lost 70 pounds in about six months, and I've kept it off for over two years now. I didn't want to lose any more than 70 pounds, so the weight loss just stopped at that point. I think the mind controls a lot of what happens.

I look younger. I feel younger. I feel more energetic, more active, and more positive about myself—more able to make my own decisions. I'm more *me*.

Once you take control of your body weight, you seem to have control over everything else. Being overweight becomes the big focus of your life. Losing the weight has put my life back into my hands, more in my control.

Jon's method is really easy to do, and the proof is in the results.

—Carole Skabe, nanny, 55

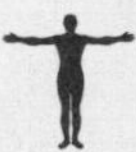

As Carole's story shows, losing weight is never just about weight loss on its own. Conrad, for example, realized that for him, the important point was an emphasis on health and life.

Conrad's Sweeter Life

In my early teens I was always carrying a little bit of weight. As I got older, I put on more weight, and when I got to 211 pounds, I started thinking that this weight is probably doing me serious damage. I started to want to pick up surfing again. So, first I read Kathleen DesMaisons' book *Potatoes Not Prozac* and learned about the effects of sugar and processed wheat flour on the metabolism, and I cut those out of my diet. I didn't lose any weight, but I did have more energy and felt much better.

Then I heard about Jon and his story. Everything he said made complete sense to me, and because he had so much background material to back up what he was saying, I decided to try what he recommended—especially with the visualizations and turning on SMART Mode, and all the information about the FAT programs. I found that, with the combination of listening to the CD in the evening, the meditation, the diet changes, and the exercise, I really started seeing results. It absolutely blew me away. It was amazing.

Most of my life I'd been focused on my weight and on my gut, and not being happy with the way I looked—about the fat, that I had to go to the gym, etc. But as I started to focus on the health, the weight loss became almost a byproduct of that. That was the revelation for me.

Before reading Jon's book, I was sleeping in and doing no exercise. Now I'm getting up at 6:00 AM, and doing half an hour of yoga or surfing.

I used to eat a huge meal at night and I'd always have seconds. Now I'm eating five smaller meals throughout the day . . . with lots of fresh, live organic food. I'm also having about 10,000 milligrams of omega-3 fish oils every day, and I'm mentally much more alert—more mentally agile—than I was before. It has made a huge difference. I'm definitely more confident in myself and in my relationship with my wife. I feel a lot more balanced without all those peaks and troughs that you get when you've got a lot of wheat and sugar in your diet.

I lost 35 pounds over eight months, and I've learned that the results come because the Gabriel Method is not a diet but a lifestyle change.

For me, it's all about "Am I happy? Is this sustainable?" And I think that anyone that wants to lose weight shouldn't go into it as a sort of instant fix. Jon mentions that. It's about the health aspect—raising your own awareness of your health as a human being. For me that's been the real revelation. It's been great. The weight loss is just a by-product.

Jon's been a real inspiration; the work that he's done on himself, the book, and the resources that he draws upon show a real dedication. If people have even half of his dedication, then they can do anything.

—Conrad Kenyon, web designer, 35

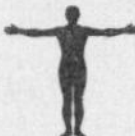

Sue was in a position that so many mothers find themselves in these days: overworked, overstressed, and with nothing left to give. Sue is another person that is near and dear to my heart. Before Sue moved down to Denmark (Australia), she was a marketing executive in Perth. After seeing me give a presentation at a local health club, she decided to take me under her wing, and she totally redesigned my book and my website. She did all this free of charge simply because she believed in what I was doing, and because she wanted to help me spread the word to the world. With her help, my book became a national bestseller in Australia within a couple of months.

I'm also so grateful to have been able to give back to her as well.

We sat down one day to talk about her weight, and I could clearly see that she was being pulled from so many directions and that she was being drained. Her weight was like a shield that she was using to keep the outside world and all of its demands at bay—a buffer between her and all of those that so desperately needed her.

Sue's story is really about reconnecting with her source.

Time for Myself

I never had much of a weight problem because I always loved exercising. Right up until three weeks before my baby was born, I was going to the gym five times a week and loving it. And I've found that whenever I've stopped exercising for any length of time for any reason, I'm just not as happy as I normally am.

It was quite a difficult birth; she was three weeks early and things weren't quite ready. I'm quite an organized person and I'm used to being efficient, and things just went all over the place. But when you're running your own business, you just have to do it. I was doing the accounts and tax reporting on the laptop from my hospital bed. The nurses couldn't believe it.

I do believe that I fell into a, well, not a post-partum depression but just a really, really hard time. I couldn't exercise because breastfeeding was every three hours, and for the first three months my baby had colic; she was just crying from early morning to about six o'clock in the evening. And my Portuguese blood makes me feel that if the house isn't clean I am even more stressed. I like to have a clean house because, if it's clean, then life's good. There was all that going on. I was so drained that there wasn't enough time to realize how drained I was, and it's really easy to get into that downward spiral.

I started having chats with Jon about how I felt really big, and he said not to worry, that after the breastfeeding stage, things should just go back to normal. But I'm such an impatient person.

Now, I was expecting Jon to talk about what I was eating and how much exercise I was doing—you know, the standard approach ... But then he asked me "What do you do to relax?" and I thought, whoa! That's a bit left of center! He said that my mind and body were reading all these things that were going on in my life like a tug-of-war and that there was "no time for you." So he wrote up this prescription. And the first thing he said was, "I want you to take one day off a week, just for yourself. I want you to put your baby into daycare, and I don't want you to do any housework or cleaning; I just want you to have that day for yourself."

And I did, but I felt really guilty because there was my husband, working really hard, and I was putting my baby into daycare. [I thought,] "Oh, God! What kind of mother am I?" But I took the day off anyway. I took Fridays off, and for the first five or six weeks after taking my prescription, I just slept the whole day. I'd drop my baby at daycare, go home, and just pass out.

Eventually though, I started taking the time out for myself, and I did go for the walks and get massages, and I guess, because I was really refilling myself, my body didn't feel deprived. It wasn't starving any more and I really didn't need the weight, so it just came off really easily, really effortlessly. I didn't have to try. I had the energy to get back to exercising again ... I got back into that mode and now I'm much happier.

Jon helped me realize that it was important that I look after myself. He also said that, at the end of the day, my husband didn't need to come home to a cranky, tired, frazzled woman because that would just put more stress on his life and on our child's. He said that if I were looked after, I could look after them better too, and that did a lot to get rid of my guilt.

Now I really feel that I'm back in balance and that, by doing the best for myself, I'm doing the best for my family too.

—Susan Correia, marketing executive and mother, 40

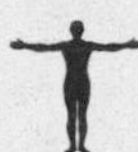

Sue ultimately lost 34 pounds in just a few months once she realized that she had to nurture herself as well as her child and husband.

Having a child is hard enough, but being pregnant and dealing with a relationship break-up at the same time—a situation that unfortunately is not all that uncommon. This the case with Gabrielle. Gabrielle Hart contacted me in August 2007 to do an interview for her radio program. During the interview, I remember her having one of those "Aha" moments, where she said, "It's all making so much sense." She called me four weeks later and said that something had completely shifted in her life. Here's her story.

Gabrielle's Magic

As a teenager, I was naturally thin. It was only really after my pregnancies that I started putting on weight. I was two months pregnant with my second child when I left my husband, and I put on a lot of weight with the stress of it all. In 2000, by the end of my second pregnancy, I'd put on about 55 pounds. I weighed about 190 pounds, then I had the baby and was down to 180. But I kept putting it back on, and going up and down. There was just this cycle. It was ridiculous, and I felt as if I was getting diabetes.

Then in October 2007, I was interviewing people for my radio program and Jon was one of them. When Jon started talking about "the feast and the famine," something just clicked. I thought "this is what I've been doing." Then he talked about the emotional reaction to a break-up, when you put the protection on, and it just made so much sense to me. All I had was the fifteen-minute interview with him, which was just amazing, and after we got off [the] air I talked with him about my situation.... In that short time we talked about my emotional eating because of my first marriage. I felt that everything had been taken from me, so I was in famine. And the second thing was that it was "safe" for me to be just that little bit overweight because then no one would feel threatened by me.

About two or three weeks later, I got the book and the CD. But even before I got the book, I lost 5 pounds. It was just this consciousness that "Oh, my goodness! My body wants to be fat!" As soon as I embraced the messages of his words, the weight just started dropping off. I didn't do anything consciously, except say to myself over and over, "I'm in feast. Wow!" And I'd go to the cupboard and see that it would always be filling up, so I could ask myself if I wanted something and then say no.

That revelation started a shift within me—just that idea that my body was doing this because it loved me—that this was the right thing to do. The minute Jon said that people are fat because their body wants to be fat, I felt a shudder go right through my body. An awakening happened. After I got the CD, I listened to it everyday. I committed to that for three-and-a-half weeks and at the end of that time, I'd lost 12 or 15 pounds. After four weeks, I had lost 22 pounds, and now a total of 34 pounds.

What's more, after those first few weeks, everything seemed to change. I found a new career path; it just opened up for me. Now, I'm all over Australia, being asked to amazing events. And the weight's just coming off—just magic beyond magic, one thing after the other.

Jon doesn't just assist you with the weight; he gets you into a state where he manages to get you to appreciate the magic of who you are and that you have something to share. And when you connect with that through his understanding, your world just opens up.

Also, my children are healthier and their concentration is up. (Gabrielle has also applied the Gabriel Method nutritional principles to her own family, even though none of them have a weight problem.) They're just better kids. And with work, I keep getting all these opportunities. They just happen. I don't have to work at it. I don't have to ask for it. I just think it's from the heart space that I'm in. The weight, the income—I'm looking younger. My skin is better. My relationship with my second husband was always fantastic, and it's even better now. It's just everything. It's like someone turned the lights on. It's like I do have magic to share, and it's safe for me to share it.

Jon helped me get out of the way and let my magic be.

—Gabrielle Hart, radio personality and performer, 37

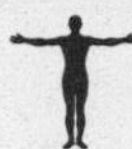

Khaliah Ali is one of the nine children (seven daughters and two sons) of former world heavyweight boxing champion Muhammad Ali. She has her own line of clothing and is involved in a lot of charity work. She's currently the Australia Zoo's Ambassador to Wildlife Warriors to the United States. Her book *Fighting Weight* (Harper Collins 2007) recounts her long struggle with obesity and her breakthrough as a result of her lap banding surgical procedure.

I thought her story was important to include because I've talked to so many people who had lap band surgery and had very disappointing results. They lost weight for a short time only to stop losing weight, or even start gaining it back. Many of them even had their bands removed. To finally get up the courage to take a measure as extreme as surgery and then to have it not work is heartbreaking. The bottom line is that whether you get surgery or not, you still have to address the real issues if you want to be successful.

Khaliah's weight loss was truly phenomenal; she lost 178 pounds in a very short time. But she attributes much of her success to the Gabriel Method. I've known Khaliah since the mid-1990s, but we connected very strongly in July 2004, when we were both the recipients of the Oneness Heart Award. I had just lost my weight, and she was scheduled to have lap band surgery the next month. We started talking on a regular basis, and I counseled her weekly while she was losing her weight. I wanted to make sure that she was adding real, live foods and omega-3s to her diet. Many people think that once they have surgery they can just drink milk shakes all day and lose weight. But what happens is their bodies go into a severe nutritional famine and this makes their body want to gain weight. She really got that, and she started to love the taste of really healthy foods. I introduced her to salads and to this day she still talks about the salad I made for her. We also talked at length about visualization and some of the real emotional issues that were at play in her life. Here's what she had to say.

Fighting from Day One

Like many overweight people, my problems came right from childhood.

I was on *The TODAY Show* for weight loss in second grade, which would put me at about eight years old and being exposed on national television for being overweight. During my twenties, I yo-yo dieted my way up from 220 to about 280. When I was approaching my thirtieth birthday, I stepped on a scale and I weighed 335 pounds. My life became crystal clear. I looked at my son, and I understood that I needed to surrender. I didn't like the way my life had been or where it was going. I was endlessly fighting my weight.

I was thirty and still very young; young enough to get my whole life together but still old enough to reflect on how much of my life I had lost. Never in my twenties had I ever sat on the beach and let the sun touch my skin. I'd never been intimate with someone completely in the buff. And also, I wanted to be healthy for my son. So much of my life was yet unlived. I had to surrender, and I needed help. I started working with Jon about a month prior to surgery, but the point of the Gabriel Method, at least to me, is that whatever path someone chooses, you're able to use the method.

The Gabriel Method actually treats a lot of the underlying causes ... that cause people to be obese and cause people to overeat. Additionally, it's filled with nutritional information and wisdom that helps people achieve optimal health.

For me there were a lot of control issues. I think that the Gabriel Method really causes you to be in the place of being—being silent and hearing what your body's telling you—perhaps for the first time in your life. When you diet, you subscribe to a lot of the things that the world has to offer, and you're taking in all the sights and sounds and belief systems of others. But with the Gabriel Method, I learned to listen to *my* voice and *my* journey.

I chose to have lap band surgery, but I also followed all of Jon's advice. I believe it was Jon's advice that enabled me to achieve truly phenomenal results. I lost over 178 pounds. I now weigh 156 pounds.

Jon's method is not a technique. He helps you get in touch with what your essential needs are as a human being—the things we've lost touch with. It's about getting in touch with what's truly right for you in your life and feeding yourself at every level of your being. His point—that most of us are starving and what we have to do is add what's missing rather than take anything away—is truly revolutionary.

How else do you explain an absolute miracle? His story is the most impressive, bar none. Very rarely do people lose so much weight. But then to maintain it and have no sagging skin is remarkable. His story is very compelling, but what's more compelling is the way he's going to go out into the world and completely transform it.

—Khaliah Ali, clothing designer, United States Ambassador to the Australia Zoo's Wildlife Warriors, 33

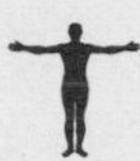

And although, as Khaliah said, for many people, age thirty is "young enough to get your whole life together," we should never see age as an impediment to transforming your life.

Consider the story of Howard, who is in his seventies and lost over forty pounds, and who has kept the weight off after decades of putting it on with too much beer and bad food. But for Howard, there's something just as important as losing the weight.

A Retired Angel Transforms

I was doing a lot of sports, including being a competitive footballer, all through my life. I joined the navy at 203 pounds when I was eighteen.

That was quality weight. I had legs like a racehorse. Even now I have a forty-six-inch chest, but after a few days eating nothing but Aussie meat pies, I'd put on another 7 pounds and I'd start getting called "tubby."

I stopped doing sports when I was thirty-three and weighed 224 pounds. And I probably drank too much after every game, which was another way to put on all those calories plus more. I just got heavier at a rate of about 5 to 7 pounds a year over twenty years or so. It wasn't a ballooning, it was just the coat was getting tighter as I was getting slacker. It wasn't that you'd notice it until you couldn't fasten the top button on your shirt. By the time I was forty-three, I was 238 pounds; by age fifty-three, I was 252 pounds.

Then there was the stress. As an accountant for some of the world's biggest companies, I had to comply with a lot of deadlines. And to keep working, I had to keep eating or drinking so that, by the morning, the work was all done. But some of my eating went into the early morning, which may have been a drink on one side and a snack on the other.

It was the wine, beer, cheese, and cookies—and peanuts. Then in the 1960s, take-out roast chickens came on the market. This was before KFC. So after a game of squash, we'd be tearing chickens apart and eating all the bad bits you aren't supposed to have these days.

I'd wanted to retire in 2000, but I had to cope with the dot com crash. I had to start work again as a real estate agent.

I hardly got a retirement. There was all that stress. It was dog eat dog.

So I attended Jon's seminar in Perth. After reading his book, I stopped drinking alcohol. He taught me that there's a thin body inside the fat body, trying to get out. Those two words "Think Thin" were the most important in the whole book. It's that. It's more than diets; it's more than the walking I do. It's the holistic side of things—getting the mind right.

I see the CD as the most essential thing. My life just changed around, and I also got a copy of *The Secret*. And now I'm just everybody's friend. Kids are coming through the front door. I've had two knee replacements, but I can walk everywhere with these poles when I couldn't do anything like that before. I'm traveling. My life has just changed so much. My whole life has gone for the better. I've had to re-tailor some clothes and give some away.

Jon certainly got me up and running. Jon Gabriel gave me that gift.

I can't see myself going backwards from here. I've got so much happiness inside of me.

—Howard Angel, retired accountant, 74

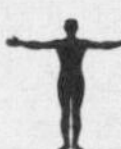

Amanda's story is truly exceptional. After I was on *A Current Affair* in May 2005, Amanda called me asking for a copy of my book. The book was nowhere near finished at that time, but Amanda never forgot me. She called me every six months, asking how the book was going. In February 2007, she called again and I sent her a complimentary copy for being so patient. I didn't know anything about her or her situation. Six months later, she called me again, but this time it was to tell me that she had lost 113 pounds and that her severe, type 2 diabetes was all but reversed. Her blood sugar levels had gone down from a life threatening seventeen to nineteen to a very healthy five to seven, and her doctor couldn't believe it. After I got off the phone with her, I thought to myself that if I never accomplish anything else in my life, there's a sixty–nine-year-old woman out there who has just been given a new lease on life. And somehow I was able to contribute to that. I felt a tremendous sense of completion, like my life and all the struggles that I had gone through were for a purpose. They were not in vain.

A New Lease on Life

I was always reasonably overweight—always a heavy-set person—even as a young girl. I was about 210 pounds. I'm a heavy-framed girl, so I never looked fat. It was after I retired that I really ballooned out. My girlfriend used to call me the Michelin Man. I put on a huge amount of weight. Just after I retired, I became broader in the shoulders, and got bigger in the boobs and the legs. It took about two years after I retired for Michelin Woman to come out. I fluctuated up and down. I tried things, but nothing ever worked.

At one point, I was working out every single night for about six months and only lost about fifteen pounds. Then if I stopped, I put everything back on in a matter of weeks. Then there was the normal fatigue that you get when you're carrying a lot of weight. You lose interest in everything because you don't want to do anything. I basically vegetated for years.

Then I saw Jon on TV and something clicked. It was like "This is your answer." I phoned up, but the book wasn't ready yet. Periodically, I'd keep calling because I was still trying to lose weight. Then in early 2007, Jon sent me the book and the CD. I still play the CD every night. I won't go to bed without playing the CD. It was like a miracle. After reading the book and listening to the CD, I just felt "this is right," and I started losing weight. At first, I didn't think too much about it, but then I started getting into shape. My daughter was the first person to notice it: I didn't have a belly that hung over my knees anymore.

I don't feel the need to eat carbohydrates, breads, cakes, and cookies. To be honest with you, I just lost interest. The CD is brilliant. I cut out a picture of a young girl with a beautiful figure and put it next to my bed to visualize it. I figured I'd focus on the major parts that I wanted to be slim: the arms, the legs, and the bum. So I listen to the CD, look at the picture, turn the light out, and go to sleep. Quite often I don't hear the end of the CD, but I sleep right through and wake up feeling good.

I've been really intuitive most of my life. I really think that when you're meant to see something, you see it, and that's why I kept pursuing the book—because I knew it was right for me. I felt that it would work, and it *did* work. I lost 113 pounds in about six months. I never really kept track of what I was losing or when I was losing it, and I didn't weigh myself or measure myself.

I have kept it off now for about eight months so far, and I'm not putting it on again. I won't stop listening to the CD. I won't stop doing my visualization every single night. The CD is my mantra.

Also, at the start, my blood sugar levels would fluctuate between sixteen and seventeen and go as high as twenty, but when I started the Gabriel Method it was about seventeen. In the last twelve months it's gone down to seven and five. I'm within the normal range. They say I still have diabetes, but I don't think I do. I don't need to worry about it.

I'm planning to learn Italian. I'd always wanted to, but when I put all the weight on I didn't want to do anything. Now I want to be part of the world again. I didn't have a social life for a long time. I didn't want to do anything or see anyone. But now! I went downhill for a long time but, because I crashed pretty quickly, I think I picked up pretty quickly. Maybe that's just the way I'm built. Now I'm able to structure my thinking in a more positive way.

—Amanda Pierce, retired call center operator, 70

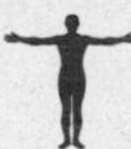

In the midst of all these stories about losing weight and changing your life, there comes the completely unexpected. As I was compiling stories for this chapter, Karen called me out of the blue just to tell me how grateful she was to me for writing the book, and how much of an impact it's had on her life. This is Karen's story.

Not Just About Losing Weight

I don't have a weight problem. I'm a naturally skinny person, but I've suffered from very serious health problems. I had severe candida and was on the anti-candida diet for four years. I'd been diagnosed with diabetes insipidis and urinary tract infections. Body-wise, I just wasn't functioning properly. I wasn't sleeping properly. I was going to the toilet two, three times a night. My bowels wouldn't work. I couldn't eat; I couldn't think. I couldn't remember. Some days I couldn't even get out of bed because my health was so bad. I could sleep for three days and still be tired. I'd been under every medical track you can imagine. I had high acidity in my blood. I had hair and nail analysis, and they found I had high mercury levels, low calcium. It didn't matter what good food I was eating, the nutrients just weren't getting to my cells.

Then my partner bought Jon's book. There are a thousand and one weight-loss books out there, and I didn't think anything of it, but then he bought all of these weight-loss supplements like digestive enzymes and the omegas and flaxseed oil and all that, and I thought "These are damn good supplements!" Then my partner lost eighteen pounds and I thought, "This guy must really know what he's talking about!"

So out of curiosity, I decided to have a look at Jon's book. Chapter 6 just blew me away because I realized I had to accept myself, my family, my upbringing, and that I had to forgive—forgive my mother, forgive my father—forgive all the bad things that ever happened to me.

The first time I read that chapter I nearly threw it across the room into the wall because I thought "You've got to be kidding! I'm NEVER going to be forgiving these people in my entire life." The second time I read it, about three months later, I played around with the idea a bit in my mind. I thought, well, maybe I could, maybe I couldn't. And I decided "No, I'm not doing it."

I thought that forgiveness was being weak. So I couldn't forgive because I had to show "them" I was strong, and that I would fight them. That was my mentality. I had to learn to be independent, so I built this big wall surrounding me. I thought that no one could get to me, that I was strong, but I was really a lost soul.

When I finished reading the book again, I started reading it again from the beginning—straight through—and I realized that I just had no choice. Forgiveness was a step I had to take because my health was getting worse and worse.

What I also realized after reading the book and listening to Jon's CD was that I was telling myself I had candida all day, every day. I'd get up in the morning and say to myself "I do this because I have candida. I can't do this because I have candida." I was telling myself this five hundred times a day and something just clicked with me. No wonder I have candida; I keep telling myself I've got it. So I just started visualizing myself being healthy—visualizing myself being candida free, telling the sickness in my body, "You're allowed to leave now. I don't need you anymore. You're free to go."

Then one day, I'd hit rock bottom. I was bawling my eyes out. I picked up Jon's book because his book always cheers me up for some reason.... I came to chapter 6 again and it cornered me. There was just no way that I would get healthier unless I embraced forgiveness.

That night I went to bed and did what he said in the book. I accepted things, went to sleep. Slept like a log, like a baby. Best sleep in my life. The first step is always the hardest; after that it was just easy. Now I have a journal with a rule that I only write positive things down. Positive words, positive thoughts I've had that day. And words about how happy I am that I'm healthy, and everything is just so much easier and lighter.

My healing was instantaneous. The whole health problem was gone within twenty-four hours. Eighty or ninety percent of my "candida" was gone overnight. My body let go. I just let it go. I honestly think that Jon is just so switched on. I dealt with a lot of people in the medical industry, and I don't trust anyone with a white coat because I feel they have just no idea what they're talking about. For some crazy reason, this naturally skinny person was drawn to Jon and his book more than anything. It made me feel good that someone understood me.

I had tried everything else in the past four years, but the Gabriel Method was the only thing that worked for me. I'm flying. I'm bulletproof now. I feel like I'm the healthiest person on this planet.

—Karen, dog groomer, 24

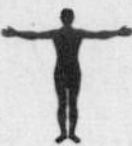

If you'd like to read the full transcripts of these stories and many others, please visit gabrielmethod.com. I'm actually thinking of turning them into book because each story is so inspiring and heart warming. And as you begin your transformation, I ask that you please keep in touch with me; feel free to call or email me anytime. I would love nothing more than to include you in that book. You can make it happen, and I am here to help you any way that I can.

It's now time to make it happen for you.

PART V

Making It Happen for You

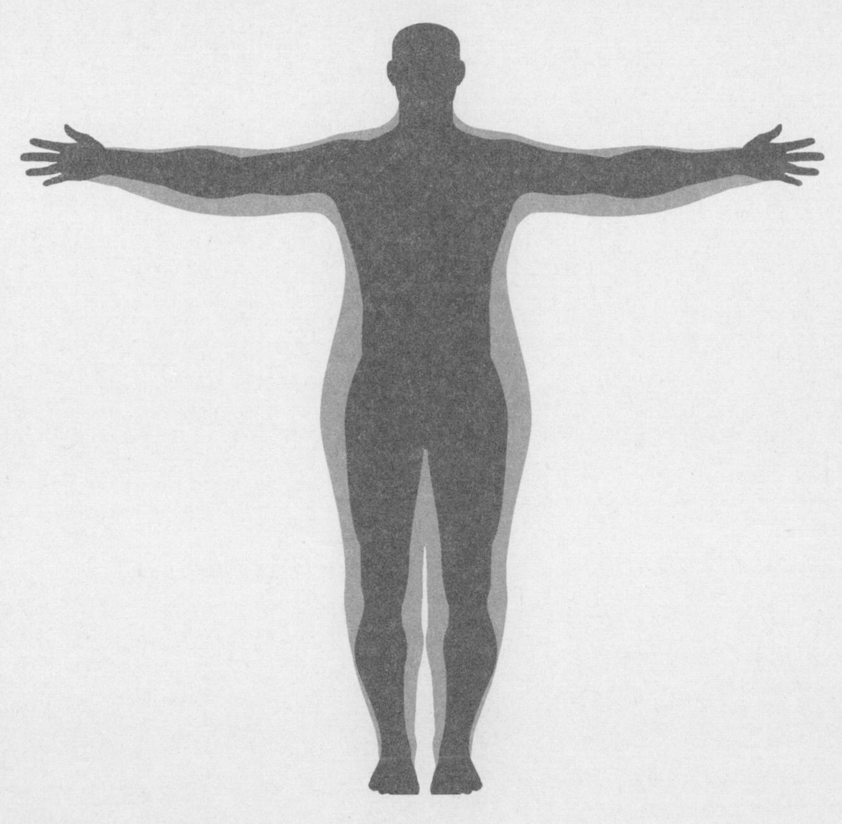

18

Creating Your New Body

Okay, let's put this all together and design an approach that works for you. As you will see, it's pretty easy to do: just focus on a few things each month until they become habits. Once they are habits, you won't have to think about them ever again.

The Approach Month by Month

Month One

At night: At night before you go to sleep, look at the picture you have selected, practice visualization for a few seconds, and then listen to the Gabriel Method CD.[1] Allow yourself to drift off to sleep while listening to the CD.

I recommend doing this every night for the first month, or several times a week at least, and then on a regular basis for the following few months. The CD addresses *all* of the many possible forms of emotional starvation, emotional obesity, and mental obesity. It also helps you practice visualization while in the highly receptive state of SMART Mode. In this way, all night long you will be creating a body that wants to be thin, while you're getting a great night's sleep.

First thing in the morning: First thing in the morning, as soon as you open your eyes, pick up the picture again, look at it, then close your eyes again and imagine yourself in perfect shape. Do this just for thirty seconds. Then imagine the rest of your day going exactly the way you would like it to go.

Breakfast: Have a great breakfast. Eat anything you want, even including the sorts of foods you'd have for dinner. If you like eating grains and potatoes (something that I am not necessarily suggesting), mornings are the best times to eat them. Just remember to go organic and whole grain whenever possible. Try to allow more time for either breakfast or lunch so you can eat somewhat leisurely. It would be terrific if you could eat one of these meals with your family so they become family meals.

Supplements

It's also important to add the following supplements:

- First thing in the morning, on an empty stomach, have a probiotic and two glasses of water (see chapter 12).
- I suggest taking at least two digestive enzyme capsules with breakfast. You can also take enzyme capsules with other meals (chapter 12).
- Take five to ten grams of an omega-3 supplement. You can take them all at once or throughout the day (chapter 10).
- I also recommend taking a multivitamin and a multimineral. Make sure your multivitamin includes vitamin E.

Afternoon Snacks

In the afternoon, have some healthy, preferably organic fruit and nuts, or any other "real" food I have recommended in this book.

Water

Drink a glass of water before each meal, before each snack, and lots of water at night (chapter 13).

Add Real Foods

Make an effort to add more live, fresh, and organic foods to your meals (chapters 10 and 15).

Month Two

Add a SMART Mode Session

If you want to take things to the next level, or as an alternative to listening to the CD, have a ten-minute SMART Mode session, preferably first thing in the morning (chapter 8).

After a few months or so, you may want to stop listening to the CD at night, but I recommend the morning visualization as a habit that you adopt for life. If your experiences are anything like mine, you may find you won't want to give up this morning session for anything. Once you have made the morning session a habit, you'll have a powerful mechanism in place for changing and improving any aspect of your life that you desire.

If you stop listening to the CD, you should still spend a moment or two practicing visualization at night and first thing in the morning.

I usually practice visualization every night for a few seconds as I am going to sleep, and it's become a habit. But there was a period of time, after I lost the weight, that I thought I didn't have to do this anymore. I thought that I had "arrived" and that I no longer needed the practice. What happened after a few weeks was that I noticed I was eating more and thinking more about food. As a result, I started to become very worried that something had changed, that my body no longer wanted to be as thin. I then resumed practicing visualization every night as before, and everything went back to normal. I started eating less and thinking less about food.

I now see the daily practice of visualization like "setting the dials on the automatic pilot." Storms and crosswinds can make a plane veer off course no matter how good the autopilot is. The stresses and strains of the daily grind can have the same effect on your body, causing it to veer off course too. When you invest thirty seconds using visualization every night, you're resetting the dials on your automatic pilot so you won't go off course.

Eat leisurely

- Focus on eating more leisurely. This month, make an effort to eat slowly and to chew your food very thoroughly. Try to get out of the habit of eating while watching TV or reading. Become a "conscious" eater.
- Turn lunch or dinner into a salad. Whatever you're eating, even if it's lasagna or a full turkey dinner, cut it up and mix it with lots of fresh greens. Put on as much salad dressing as you like, and use a salad dressing that you really love. Make the salad something that tastes great and is very satisfying.
- Take a short break after eating for five or ten minutes to give your brain a chance to catch up with your stomach, and to send the message that food is abundant and there is no need to rush.
- Stop as soon as you feel full, even if you're just stopping for a minute or two. You can always start eating again whenever you like (chapter 15).

Month Three

Enhance Your Life Force

Add a ten-minute Super-Vitality Break, either first thing in the morning or in the early afternoon (chapter 15).

- Have a shot of fresh wheatgrass juice if possible. If wheatgrass is not available, have some other source of live chlorophyll, like fresh spinach or any other dark, leafy greens.
- Spend at least five minutes outside in nature, practicing the Eating the Sun technique or just walking around somewhere peaceful and quiet—beside a stream or in a park (chapter 11).

Shift Your Body's Hunger Habit

- Make an effort this month to eat more of your food during the day, late afternoon, and early evening. Over time, you'll

train your body to be hungrier during the day and less so at night. Eventually, your body will be in the habit of eating and being hungry when you actually need the food, instead of storing it all night (chapter 15).
- Remember to drink lots of water at night, as drinking will kill nighttime hunger pangs.

Eat When You Are Hungry, Not When You Are Programmed to Eat

While it's important to eat a large breakfast and, in the beginning, "real" snacks in the afternoon, if you find you're not hungry at dinner, don't eat just because it's dinner. There is no rule that says we absolutely have to eat at mealtimes. Now that you are adding more food and *healthier* food earlier in the day, if you're not hungry at night, that is the greatest thing possible. The absence of hunger at night is your body's way of telling you that it wants to lose weight. Let it happen.

Of course, if you're going out with family and friends, eat and enjoy yourself. But on those occasions when you're not going out, or there is nothing special planned and you're not hungry, allow yourself to lose weight. Go with what your body wants; you can eat whenever and you whatever you want. Don't eat just because you are conditioned to do so.

This is something that "naturally thin" people do; they skip a lot of meals. We always focus on all the food naturally thin people eat, but we never pay attention to all the times they don't eat. They are not eating simply because their bodies are not hungry. So if you're going to eat like a naturally thin person, then *don't eat* like one as well.

Month Four
Activate the "Get Thin or Get Eaten" Adaptation

- By now, your body has been changing for several months. It no longer wants to be fat. You'll have much more energy and may have had it for some time. You may want to start to experiment with living a more outdoorsy, active, sporty lifestyle, and see if it agrees with you. You may find that you get hooked on something and it becomes one of the highlights of your life.

- Practice the visualizations discussed in chapter 16 for loving exercise and for maximizing its benefits.
- Add some good stresses that will cause your body to want to be thin—anything that is thrilling or exciting that you have been wanting to do (chapter 16).
- Turn a bad stress into a good stress. When you are experiencing stress at work or at any other time, get up and move (chapter 16)!

Use Visualization to Kill Junk Food Addictions

Visualization is very effective for eliminating the desire to eat junk food. Once you eliminate the desire, eliminating the food becomes like releasing an anchor. This enables you to get all the weight-loss benefits of eating properly without any of the mental, emotional, or biochemical drawbacks to dieting.

If at this point you still have any lingering junk food addictions, try practicing this visualization technique. It's quick, it's easy, and it's painless. It is also extremely effective.

The Killing the Craving Technique

Technique: All you have to do is to imagine yourself eating something that you would like to stop eating, and then imagine something repulsive happening while you're eating the food.

Since everyone is different, you have to decide what you find repulsive.

Maggots repulse me. So what I used to do is imagine that I was eating a piece of bread when all of a sudden I noticed that it was laced with maggots. I could see them wiggling around on the bread, and I could feel them moving around in my mouth. I then imagined spitting out the food, and becoming nauseated and disgusted.

That's all you have to do. You imagine a negative experience, and by doing so, create a negative association with the particular food you wish to eliminate. However, the key to making the negative association stay with you for life is making the association while you are in SMART Mode (chapter 5).

In SMART Mode, you become as impressionable as a child. A friend of mine used to come over from time to time, and I would always make something for him to eat. I noticed that he always had an excuse for not eating whatever I had prepared. Finally, I confronted him on the matter, and he said that once when he was a kid, one of his friends prepared a sandwich for him and, as a joke, the friend had secretly spat in it.

His friend eventually told him about it after he had eaten the sandwich. This incident left such an indelible impression on his mind that for thirty years he has never been able to eat anything if one of his friends has prepared it. Think of how many meals he has missed over the last thirty years because of that one chance incident. That's what can happen when you have a negative experience like this as a child.

In SMART Mode, your brain can't differentiate between real and imagined experiences, so when you visualize in SMART Mode, your brain really and truly believes that it's actually happening. So, when working to kill a craving, the more negative the better! And the more personally offensive the association, the more useful it will be.

One woman once told me that mussels made her nauseous because, as a child, she ate a bad one and got food poisoning. So I told her to imagine mussels on the food. This worked very well for her.

It's also useful if there is something repulsive that the food resembles. For example, sugar looks like ground glass. You can imagine eating a sugar-coated doughnut and discovering that it's laced with ground glass—glass that is cutting you up inside. Another woman told me that after making this association, she could not even walk by a bakery without feeling nauseous.

Chocolate is also an easy one because chocolate looks like so many repulsive things, like dirt or mud or things that are too offensive to mention. The more repulsive the scene, the greater the impression will be in your mind. So if you imagine that you are eating some chocolate ice cream, for example, only to find—after it's too late—that it's one of those more offensive things, you may never be able to look at chocolate again!

Once you have practiced the visualization in SMART Mode a few times, you can practice it during the day in your normal waking state and get the same result. Whenever you see the food during the day and you are craving it, replay the visualization in your mind and you will quickly become repulsed.

The time to practice this technique, if you need to at all, is *after you have spent a few months removing the reasons your body wants to be fat.* Most likely, you will not need to use this technique at all since you will just start to crave less junk food automatically. However, if you ever want to use the "Kill the Craving" technique, it works quickly, and it's worked for everyone that I've introduced it to.

Using my approach, you never actually give up a food through will power; you *eliminate the craving* for it instead.

Going Forward

Finally, as you are transforming your body, FOLLOW YOUR HEART.

If there is anything that your heart is calling out for you to experience, listen to it, trust it, and take the chance.

See Yourself Being Thin All Day

Whenever you think about it during the day, visualize yourself being thin. No matter what you're doing, take the opportunity to imagine you are doing it with a thin, "ideal" body.

Time of Day	MONTH ONE
Just before bed	Look at the picture Visualize: Your ideal body *Two minutes*
Just after that	Listen to the CD as you are falling asleep
First thing in the morning, while lying in bed	Visualize: Your ideal body *Two minutes*
Before breakfast	Drink two glasses of water with a probiotic
Breakfast	Have a large breakfast Add protein; omega-3; fresh, live food & digestive enzymes

Time of Day	MONTH TWO
Lunch	Eat leisurely Add any salad you love
Afternoon snack	Add something "real"
Sometime during the day	A *ten-minute* SMART Mode visualization session (best in morning)
Supplements	Omega-3 Multivitamin and Multimineral Add "real" foods when possible
Water	Before meals and snacks, at night, and whenever thirsty

Time of Day	MONTH THREE
Just before bed	Visualize: 1. Your ideal body 2. Having a Super-Vitality Break the next day *Two minutes*
Just after that	Listen to a weight-loss CD if you still want to
First thing in the morning, while lying in bed	Visualize: 1. Your ideal body 2. Visualize the coming day *One minute*
Before breakfast	Drink two glasses of water with a probiotic
Breakfast	Have a large breakfast Add protein; omega-3; fresh, live food & digestive enzymes
Lunch	Have a large lunch with real food and shift your hunger habit by eating more in the late afternoon
Afternoon	Super-Vitality Break (*ten minutes*)
Afternoon snack	Add something "real" Eat more during the daytime
Dinner	Eat earlier if possible Drink extra water at night
Sometime during the day	A *ten-minute* SMART Mode visualization session (best in the morning)
Supplements	Omega-3 Multivitamin and Multimineral Add "real" foods when possible
Water	Before meals and snacks, at night, and whenever thirsty

Time of Day	MONTH FOUR
Just before bed	Visualize: 1. Your ideal body 2. Being physically active the next day *Two minutes*
Just after that	Listen to the CD periodically as needed
First thing in the morning, while lying in bed	Visualize: 1. Your ideal body 2. Being physically active *One minute*
Before breakfast	Drink two glasses of water with a probiotic
Breakfast	Have a large breakfast Add protein; omega-3; fresh, live food & digestive enzymes
Lunch	Continue to shift your hunger habit by eating more during the day
Afternoon	Super-Vitality Break (*ten minutes*)
Dinner	Eat earlier if possible Drink extra water at night
Sometime during the day	A *ten-minute* SMART Mode visualization session (best in the morning)
Supplements	Omega-3 CLA Multivitamin and Multimineral Add "real" foods when possible
Sometime during the day	Reconnect with being physically active Do something that you enjoy Rest at least three days in a week
Water	Before meals and snacks, at night, and whenever thirsty

Time of Day	GOING FORWARD
Just before bed	Visualize: 1. Your ideal body 2. Your ideal life *One minute*
First thing in the morning, while lying in bed	Visualize: 1. Your ideal body 2. Your ideal life *One minute*
Sometime during the day	Continue the positive habits that you have acquired
Some final advice	Live an active, vibrant life TRUST YOUR HEART AND FOLLOW IT

NOTE:

1. Please go to http://www.gabrielmethod.com/cd for instructions on how to download *The Gabriel Method Evening Visualization* CD for free.

19

How Quickly Will I Lose the Weight?

As you know by now, the Gabriel Method is not a diet. The allure of all diets is how quickly you'll lose weight. But no one ever talks about the rebound effect that happens when you go off the diet. The Gabriel Method is not a diet—it's not something you are on again, off again. It is not even a program really. It's a concept and an approach. The concept is straightforward: as long as your body wants to be fat, it will *force you to be fat*, and when your body wants to be thin, it will *force you to be thin*. The approach is geared towards eliminating the reasons why your body wants to be fat and solving your problems forever. How quickly you will lose weight depends on your particular circumstances.

If obesity has been a lifetime struggle for you and you've had a long history of dieting, it will take some time to undo the hormonal and chemical issues as well as the mental and emotional ones. Most likely, your body has lost the ability to burn fat efficiently. The ability to burn fat takes time to regain. You may lose weight slowly at first or not at all.

In fact, in the first few weeks, you may actually gain weight as a rebound from coming out of chronic starvation caused by years of dieting and depriving yourself.

After a few weeks, however, you'll find that while you're eating whatever you want, the types of food you crave are much healthier and you just don't think about food as much. When that happens, you'll start to lose weight consistently.

Then something truly incredible happens. As you eliminate the reasons your body thinks it needs to be fat, you'll start losing weight faster and faster. When your body wants to be thin, it becomes very efficient at burning fat; it becomes a fat burning machine. The thinner your body wants to be, the faster you will lose weight. For this reason, the rate at which you're losing weight can actually accelerate right up to the very end.

This is not to say that you will not experience plateaus. You should expect to reach some plateaus, but if you measure the rate at which you lose weight, over time you'll find that you are losing weight faster.

Once you have lost the weight you would like to lose, you'll easily be able to maintain your ideal weight because there is no diet or program that you have been on that you will now want to discontinue; you haven't been depriving yourself. You've just been transforming your body by making it *want* to be and *need* to be thin. In doing so, you'll have acquired positive eating and lifestyle habits that will last a lifetime.

Fast and Loose

Another great reason to lose weight this way is that your skin will be tighter after the weight is gone. When you try to force yourself to lose weight quickly by crash dieting or surgery, you can end up with excessively loose skin. This is because the stress of forcing yourself to lose weight elevates your cortisol levels, and cortisol causes your skin to lose its elasticity. The Gabriel Method is a low-stress way to lose weight that helps lower your cortisol levels and keeps your skin as elastic as possible.

The detoxifying, rejuvenating, and revitalizing aspects of my approach will also help your skin respond well to weight loss—as will visualization. In fact, everything about losing weight this way will help ensure that, after the weight is gone, your skin is healthier, more firm, vibrant, and elastic.

So, for all these reasons, the focus should never be on how fast you lose weight; the focus should always be on eliminating the whole "fat" issue entirely and creating the body of your dreams.

Starting Tonight

Getting started is easy, and you can start as soon as tonight. First, download the Gabriel Method CD. Then do some visualization as you are going to sleep. In addition to visualizing your ideal body, visualize going to the store tomorrow and picking up some of the items you will need for month one.

Month One Checklist

- A picture of your ideal body
- Probiotics
- Digestive enzymes
- Multivitamins and multiminerals
- Omega-3 supplements
- Fresh produce—preferably locally grown, in season, and organic

See my website for the Super Delicious, Super Nutritious recipes and other items you may want to pick up, such as flaxseeds, flaxseed oil, whey protein, and xylitol.

If you take the first step tonight, you will have done the hardest thing that you will need to do—overcome inertia. Once you overcome the inertia, a positive momentum develops in your life, and you will be well on your way to transforming your body—and maybe even your life.

It can all happen with one simple step—starting tonight!

Download the
Gabriel Method Evening Visualization CD
for free at
http://www.gabrielmethod.com/cd

Appendix: The Chemistry of the FAT Programs

This appendix is primarily for those readers who have a scientific background or who have a scientific orientation. It presumes some prior knowledge of biochemistry.

"FAT Programs" is a term that I use for a metabolic profile that can cause a shift in the body's internal "set-point," signaling to the body that it needs to be fatter for reasons of self-preservation and survival.

Leptin and the Internal Set-Point

Leptin is a hormone produced by our fat cells. Among other things, it communicates to the brain how much fat our bodies are carrying.

Since its discovery in 1994, the role of leptin has radically altered the field of metabolic physiology. Leptin is widely considered to be the master hormone that regulates body weight. It causes feelings of satiety,[1] reduces sugar cravings,[2] signals the thyroid to speed up the metabolism,[3] and signals to the liver to start burning fat.[4]

The net effect is that when leptin levels rise, we eat less, we burn more calories, and we burn fat very easily. It is for this reason that, when leptin was discovered back in 1994, it was thought to have the potential to solve the obesity epidemic.

Rats were genetically altered so that they were incapable of producing leptin. These rats remained insatiably hungry and eventually grew to be three times their normal weight.[5] Administering leptin to these rats caused them to lose weight in a dose-dependent fashion: the more leptin they were given, the thinner they became.[6] A rare genetic defect in humans that causes a deficiency in leptin also causes severe obesity, and is effectively treated with leptin.[7]

Unfortunately, the enthusiasm for leptin quickly abated because, with the exception of those rare few who did have this leptin genetic defect, administering leptin to obese people had little or no effect. Nearly all obese individuals already have elevated leptin levels, simply because the fatter one is, the more leptin their fat cells will produce. The problem with chronically obese people is not that they have too little leptin, but the fact that they have become insensitive to it. Their bodies aren't listening to leptin, and the relevant cells are not responding to or reacting to leptin as they should. The technical term for this chemical deafness is "leptin resistance."

The net effect of leptin resistance is the same as having little or no leptin. The worse the leptin resistance, the fatter someone will become.

The answer is not in more leptin but in getting your body to start listening to leptin again, or becoming more sensitive to leptin. The more sensitive you are to leptin, the thinner you'll become.

Leptin-sensitive people:

- Are less hungry
- Feel satiated very quickly
- Crave fewer sugary foods
- Have faster metabolisms
- Have more energy
- Retain the ability to burn fat efficiently

So the real key to determining how fat or thin one will be lies in how sensitive or resistant his or her body is to leptin.

Your Body's Set-Point

Many researchers believe that leptin plays a dominant role in managing your body's "internal set-point." The internal set-point theory asserts that your body has an ideal weight it wants to be and it will seek to maintain that weight. If your weight exceeds your body's set-point, you'll become less hungry and eat less until your body weight falls back down to its set-point level. If your body weight falls below the set-point, you'll become hungry and eat more until your body weight achieves the desired set-point level again.

Many people who believe in an internal set-point take a fatalistic view that it's a number that cannot be altered. However, it makes more sense that the level of our internal set-point is determined not only by genetics but also by environmental and emotional stress factors—so our internal set-point shifts, depending upon the survival stresses we have in our lives.

One study conducted by Dallman et al strongly supports the notion that our internal set-point is largely dependent upon stress.[8] In this study, researchers hooked up rats to electrodes that bioelectrically simulated the chronic, low-level stress of the modern human experience. The rats then had a choice of eating their normal food or high-calorie food, and drinking regular water or sugar water.

The stressed rats chose higher calorie food and sugar water over their normal diet. They also gained a substantial amount of weight. The control rats chose their normal diet and did not gain any weight. Furthermore, when the electrodes were removed from the rats, they went back to eating their usual diet, and their weight eventually returned to normal. The stress had temporarily shifted their internal set-point, and when the stress was removed, their set-point shifted back.

I believe that our internal set-point determines our sensitivity to leptin. Whenever your body shifts its set-point, all it has to do to enforce this shift is simply adjust its sensitivity level to leptin. If your body decides for survival reasons that your internal set-point should shift toward being fatter, you'll become leptin resistant. Anytime your body decides it is more advantageous to be thinner, it will become more sensitive to leptin. It's really a very simple and elegant program.

In this book, when I say that "the body has activated the FAT Programs," what I mean is that the internal set-point has shifted towards being fatter, and consequently, the relevant areas of the brain and body have become more leptin resistant.

FAT Program Triggers

The question then becomes, what causes our set-point to shift and what causes our bodies to become more or less sensitive to leptin? In other words, what controls the FAT Programs?

There are a number of chemical and hormonal signals that can cause or influence leptin resistance. Among them are:

- Chronically elevated cortisol levels (either plasma cortisol[9] levels or intracellularly, in adipose tissue[10])
- Elevated triglycerides[11]
- Insulin resistance[12]
- Proinflammatory cytokines, such as tumor necrosis factor-alpha (TNF-alpha), Interluken-6, and c-reactive protein[13]

Cortisol and Leptin Resistance

The relationship between cortisol and leptin resistance is undeniable. A condition called Cushing's Syndrome causes chronically elevated levels of cortisol in the blood stream. People who suffer from Cushing's Syndrome are characteristically obese and have leptin resistance.[14] Similarly, people who take medication which artificially elevates cortisol levels are also characteristically obese and have leptin resistance. However, when they stop taking the medication, the situation reverses.

The relationship between cortisol and leptin resistance goes even further. Adrenalectimized rats have no adrenal glands and are incapable of producing cortisol. These rats do not easily get fat nor will they become leptin resistant. Administering cortisol intravenously to adrenalectimized rats will cause them to gain weight and to become leptin resistant in a dose-dependent fashion.[15] That is, the more cortisol they are given over time, the fatter and more leptin resistant they will become.

While the relationship between cortisol and leptin resistance is widely acknowledged, it is frequently discounted. The reasons being that most overweight people do not have significantly elevated cortisol levels. However, the relationship between elevated cortisol levels and leptin resistance extends beyond plasma cortisol levels.

Cortisol levels can be elevated intracellularly. Elevated cortisol levels within the cells may not show up in a blood, saliva, or urine test, causing professionals to discount this relationship too quickly. The 11-beta-hydroxysteroid-dehydrogenase-1 enzyme (11-BHSD-1), present in some fat, liver, and brain cells, converts inactive cortisone to active cortisol, increasing the cortisol levels inside the cell.[16] The over expression of the 11-BHSD-1 enzyme can cause a kind of intracellular hypercortisolism.

Studies have shown the 11-BHSD-1 enzyme is very active in the fat cells of most obese people.[17] Studies with mice have also demonstrated that, when this enzyme is overly active, obesity and leptin resistance will result.[18] What causes the body to activate this enzyme is a question that many experts are now trying to answer. Researchers today, backed by substantial funding, are targeting this enzyme as a potential obesity treatment. Because of this enzyme, many people are now calling central obesity "Cushing's Syndrome of the fat cells."[19]

Leptin Resistance and Triglycerides

An interesting study conducted in 2004 showed that triglycerides can cause a type of leptin resistance by binding to leptin in the blood stream and preventing it from crossing the blood–brain barrier.[20]

As a result, the brain gets an inaccurate assessment of the actual amount of leptin that is circulating in the blood stream. Since many of the leptin receptors in the brainstem exist before the blood–brain barrier, this is clearly not the only mechanism at play. Nonetheless, it would certainly have some affect on the brain's energy homeostasis regulation and could easily cause a set-point shift.

Insulin Resistance and Leptin Resistance

Insulin resistance and leptin resistance are also highly correlated in obesity. While leptin resistance can cause insulin resistance, the reverse may also be true. Studies have shown that insulin can activate the expression of the suppressor of the cytokine signaling 3 (SOCS3) gene in certain cells.[21] Activating the SOCS3 in the arcuate and paraventrical nucleus of the hypothalamus can cause leptin resistance by preventing downstream signaling.

Insulin resistance leads to hyperinsulinemia, or chronically elevated insulin levels. Hyperinsulinemia could then possibly cause leptin resistance. It is interesting to note that chronically elevated cortisol levels, both plasma and intracellular, can cause elevated triglycerides and insulin resistance.[22]

Proinflammatory Cytokines and Leptin Resistance

TNF-A and IL-6 have been shown to both activate the expression of the 11-BHSD-1 enzyme in certain fat cells[23] and cause insulin resistance.[24] They may also increase the expression of the SOCS3 gene in certain cells.[25]

The Metabolic Profile of Obesity

Nearly all obese people are leptin resistant, and they characteristically have elevated cortisol levels (either serum or intracellular), elevated triglycerides, insulin resistance, and hyperinsulinemia. The proinflammatory cytokines mentioned are also considered biomarkers for obesity.

The Famine and Temperature Stress Response and Obesity

Starvation and cold weather are environmental stresses that favor the accumulation and preservation of fat for survival reasons. Chronic exposure to starvation and/or cold weather should, in theory, make the body want to be fatter and cause the internal set-point to shift. In fact, studies support this notion. For example, rats exposed to cold weather for the first two months of their life grow to be heavier than normal as adults.[26] This indicates that the chronic exposure to cold weather caused their internal set-point to shift. Interestingly, a study of over four thousand women in Britain found that those born during the coldest months of the winter were more likely to have insulin resistance and elevated triglycerides later in life.[27]

In many ways, both starvation and the exposure to cold weather create a metabolic profile that is similar to modern day obesity. Specifically, the stress of starvation and cold temperatures causes elevated cortisol levels, both plasma[28] and intracellular, through increased expression of the 11-BHSD-1,[29] as well as elevated triglycerides[30] and insulin resistance.[31]

In the presence of these stresses, the body is clearly sending chemical signals that cause it to become more leptin resistant.

The above chemical changes that can cause or contribute to leptin resistance are part of what I consider to be a unique stress response to starvation and cold weather. As a result, our bodies are programmed to react to these signals by becoming leptin resistant. These chemical signals communicate to our bodies that we are either starving or, for some other reason, it is in our best interest to be fatter, so our set-point shifts accordingly.

Today, we experience chronically elevated cortisol, triglyceride, and proinflammatory cytokine levels, as well as insulin resistance and hyperinsulinemia from any number of environmental and emotional stresses that are completely unique to modern day life.

What could very well be happening is that the stresses of modern living are creating the same metabolic profile as perpetual starvation and/or cold weather, thus tricking our bodies into activating ancient survival mechanisms that cause our set-point to shift toward fat accumulation.

When this chemical profile is present, the body reacts as if it is starving despite the presence of unlimited food. Having the starvation stress response activated in the presence of unlimited food is a scenario our bodies have never encountered or anticipated before.

A vicious cycle then ensues. High levels of leptin also cause leptin resistance, so the fatter you get, the more leptin resistant you become. Insulin resistance, in the presence of unlimited food, causes hyperinsulinemia. Hyperinsulinemia causes the body to become extremely efficient at making fat and becoming resistant to burning fat, since insulin activates lipogenic (fat producing) enzymes and suppresses glucagon and lipolytic (fat utilization) enzymes.

I call this metabolic profile the "Famine And Temperature" stress response or the FAT stress response.

Fight or FAT

There is a difference between the "fight or flight" response and the FAT stress response.

For obvious reasons, the FAT stress response is diametrically opposed to the fight or flight stress response as far as leptin is concerned. The stress of running away from a predator should cause the body to adapt by wanting to be as lean as possible to minimize the risks associated with future attacks. The activation of the fight or flight response should, in theory, cause the set-point to shift in the opposite direction and, therefore, cause increased leptin sensitivity (as opposed to leptin resistance). The fact that acute stresses, such as exercise, lead to reduced cortisol and triglyceride levels, as well as increased insulin sensitivity, strongly supports this notion.

The fight or flight response is the common term for the stress response known as the Hypothalamus Pituitary Adrenal axis (HPA axis). Very possibly, the determining factor as to how the body will adapt to a given stress—as far as leptin is concerned—is whether or not the stress response is initiated in the hypothalamus by the release of corticotropin releasing hormone (CRH).

In the typical fight or flight response, CRH levels are elevated[32] and this initiates the HPA axis. This type of stress response will not cause chronically elevated cortisol levels since a negative feedback loop exists between cortisol and CRH. Also, CRH has been shown to increase leptin sensitivity,[33] and CRH has been associated with loss of appetite and the anorexic effect of treadmill running.[34] So the traditional fight or flight response to stress can make the body thinner, as we might expect.

However, if the stress response bypasses the hypothalamus and CRH, you lose the negative feedback loop and can have an unregulated cortisol cascade. Examples of stress responses that cause an unregulated cortisol cascade include: the "chronic stress-response network," where the amygdale produces ACTH, such as with Dallman's rats[35]; an overly active pituitary, as in Cushing's Syndrome; and the over expression of the 11-BHSD-1 enzyme. All of these stress responses have been shown to cause obesity.

Significantly, studies on starvation reveal a similar kind of stress response. While cortisol levels are elevated from food deprivation, CRH levels are reduced[36,37] or unchanged.[38] Cortisol levels are evidently being elevated through some mechanism other than CRH initiating the HPA axis.

In addition, levels of CRH-BP, a hormone that *inhibits* the action of CRH, have also been shown to be elevated in both starvation and obesity in rats.[39] So, in both obesity and starvation, the stress response is not the "normal" HPA axis/fight or flight response.

Obesity is often characterized by an "abnormal" functioning of the HPA axis. But it is possible that it is not really abnormal, just a different stress response—a starvation or "FAT" stress response, not a fight or flight response.

Mental and Emotional Stress

People generally assume that our bodies' catch-all response to mental and emotional stresses is the fight or flight response, the rationale being that the body interprets all mental and emotional threats to be some type of predator. But this assumption seems overly simplistic and is completely unfounded, as well as unprovable.

Our bodies, no doubt, interpret all mental and emotional stress as some type of physical threat. But who is to say what type of physical threat? Our bodies could be interpreting the stress to be a predator, starvation, cold weather, or any other type of physical threat.

Starvation and cold weather have their own unique stress responses. They are stresses, but they are clearly not fight or flight stresses. Your body should react differently to the threat of a predator than to the threat of starvation. Theoretically, the appropriate adaptive responses to these two threats are antagonistic in nature.

To say that your body is interpreting one type of emotional stress to be the threat of starvation is no less credible than to say that your body is interpreting the stress to be that of a predator. Both notions are based on the same fundamental, theoretical idea that our bodies perceive emotional stresses to be physical threats. The question has not been investigated thoroughly. And, in any event, given the nature of the question, it is largely unanswerable at present.

However, if mental stresses can activate the fight or flight response, it is not unreasonable to assume they can also activate the FAT stress response. Both are programmed responses to physical threats. Therefore, they should be the body's programmed response to imagined threats as well.

This offers a much more plausible explanation as to why emotional stress can cause weight gain in some instances and weight loss in others. Doctors and researchers frequently blame stress for sudden and drastic fluctuations in weight. The exact same emotional stress might lead to morbid obesity in one person and anorexia in another.

The explanation that your body is simply interpreting the stress one way versus another is a much clearer one than the typical explanations, such as a breakdown in the proper functioning of the HPA axis due to exhaustion, or the chronic activation of the HPA axis causing cortisol to stay in the blood stream longer.

A more logical explanation is that different stresses in different people cause different stress responses. In the example of anorexia, the body is interpreting the stress as a constant attack by a predator one must escape from, resulting in extreme leptin sensitivity. At the other extreme of obesity, the body is interpreting the stress to be chronic, extreme starvation or cold weather. This gives a little more credit to the body's ability to attempt to understand and differentiate one type of mental or emotional threat from another.

The issue then of how your body is interpreting the stress becomes of paramount importance. This takes us to the mind–body connection, an area of scientific study that's very much in its infancy. So many of the issues that the mind–body connection raises are likely to remain in the domain of speculation for the foreseeable future.

NOTES

1. See J. Freidman and J. Halaas, "Leptin and the Regulation of Body Weight in Mammals," *Nature* 395 (Nature Publishing Group, October 22, 1998): 763–770.

2. See H. Miura, K. Kawai, K. Nakashima, K. Sugimoto, and Y. Ninomiya, "Leptin is a Modulator of Sweet Taste Sensitivities in Mice," *Proceedings of the National Academy of Sciences of the United States of America* 97, no. 20 (September 26, 2000): 11044–11049.

3. See A. Magnano, D. Bloomfield, D. Gallagher, E. Murphy, L. Mayer, L. Weimer, M. Rosenbaum, R. Goldsmith, R. L. Leibel, and S. Heymsfield, "Low-dose Leptin Reverses Skeletal Muscle, Autonomic, and Neuroendocrine Adaptations to Maintenance of Reduced Weight," *The Journal of Clinical Investigation* 115, no 12 (American Society for Clinical Investigation, December 2005): 3579–3586.

4. See J. Friedman, "Research Identifies Enzyme Involved in Fat Storage" Howard Hughes Medical Institute Research Website (July 12, 2002): http://www.hhmi.org/news/friedman4.html.

5. See note 1 above.

6. Ibid.

7. Ibid.

8. See F. Gomez, H. Houshyar, K. Laugero, M. Bell, M. Dallman, N. Pecoraro, S. Akana, S. Bhatnagar, S. La Fleur, and S. Manalo, "Chronic Stress and Obesity: A New View of 'Comfort Food,'" *Proceedings of the National Academy of Sciences of the United States of America* 100, no. 20 (September 26, 2000): 11696–11701.

9. See G. D. Chusney, J. C. Pickup, and M. B. Mattock, "The Innate Immune Response and Type 2 Diabetes: Evidence that Leptin is Associated with a Stress-Related (Acute-Phase) Reaction," *Clinical*

Endocrinology 52, no. 1 (Society for Clinical Endocrinology, January 2000): 107–112.

10. Via the activation of the 11-HHSD-1 enzyme, which converts inactive cortisone to cortisol in certain cells.

11. See A. B. Coon, A. Moinuddin, J. E. Morley, J. M. Shultz, R. Nakaoke, S. M. Robinson, and W. A. Banks, "Triglycerides Induce Leptin Resistance at the Blood-Brain Barrier," *Diabetes* 53, no. 5 (American Diabetes Association, May 2004): 1253–1260.

12. See B. Emanuelli, C. Filloux, D. Hilton, E. Van Obberghen, and P. Peraldi, "Insulin Induces Suppressor of Cytokine Signaling-3 Tyrosine Phosphorylation through Janus-Activated Kinase," *Journal of Biological Chemistry* 276, no. 27 (American Society for Biochemistry and Molecular Biology, July 6, 2001): 24614–24620.

13. See B. Wisse, "The Inflammatory Syndrome: The Role of Adipose Tissue Cytokines in Metabolic Disorders Linked to Obesity," *Journal of the American Society of Nephrology* 15, no. 11 (November 2004): 2792–2800.

14. See H. Katner, L. Kirk, R. Hash, and T. Jones, "Cushing's Disease: Clinical Manifestations and Diagnostic Evaluation," *American Family Physician* 62, no. 5 (American Academy of Family Physicians, September 2001).

15. See A. Sainsbury, B. Jeanrenaud, F. Rohner-Jeanrenaud, I. Cusin, and K. E. Zakrzewska, "Glucocorticoids as Counterregulatory Hormones of Leptin: Toward an Understanding of Leptin Resistance," *Diabetes*, 46, no. 4 (American Diabetes Association, April 1997): 717–719.

16. See I. J. Bujalska, P. M. Stewart, and S. Kumar, "Does Central Obesity Reflect Cushing's Disease of the Omentum?" *The Lancet* 349, no. 9060 (Elsevier, April 26, 1997): 1210–1213.

17. B. R. Walker, "We Can Cure Cushing's Syndrome, So Can We Cure the Metabolic Syndrome?" *Society of Endocrinology Annual Meeting London, UK (2001)*," Endocrine Abstracts Website: http://www.endocrine-abstracts.org/ea/0002/ea0002sp9.htm.

18. Espindola-Antunes, Daniela and Kater, Claudio E. "Adipose Tissue Expression of 11ß-Hydroxysteroid Dehydrogenase Type 1 in Cushing's Syndrome and in Obesity," *Arquivos Brasileiros de Endocrinologia & Metabologia* 51, no. 8 (November 2007): 1397–1403.

19. See note 16.

20. See note 11.

21. See note 12.

22. See T. Reinehr and W. Andler, "Cortisol and Its Relation to Insulin Resistance Before and After Weight Loss in Obese Children," *Hormone Research* 62, no. 3 (Karger, 2004): 107–112.

23. See A. Strain, C. Burt, I. Bujalska, J. Moore, J. Tomlinson, M. Cooper, M. Hewison, M. Shahmanesh, and P. Stewart, "Regulation of Expression of 11ß-Hydroxysteroid Dehydrogenase Type 1 in Adipose Tissue: Tissue-Specific Induction by Cytokines," *Endocrinology* 142, no. 5 (The Endocrine Society, May 2001): 1982–1989.

24. See C. Lang, D. Dobrescu, and G. Bagby, "Tumor Necrosis Factor Impairs Insulin Action on Peripheral Glucose Disposal and Hepatic Glucose Output," *Endocrinology* 130, no. 1 (The Endocrine Society, January 1992): 43–52.

25. See C. Bjørbæk, H. Shi, I. Tzameli, and J. Flier, "Suppressor of Cytokine Signaling 3 is a Physiological Regulator of Adipocyte Insulin Signaling" *Journal of Biological Chemistry* 279, no. 33 (American Society for Biochemistry and Molecular Biology, August 13, 2004): 34733–34740.

26. See C. White, D. Braymer, D. York, and G. Bray, "Effect of a High or Low Ambient Perinatal Temperature on Adult Obesity in Osborne-Mendel and S5B/Pl Rats," *American Journal of Physiology—Regulatory, Integrative, and Comparative Physiology* 288 (American Physiological Society, 2005): R1376–R1384.

27. See D. Lawlor, G. Smith, R. Mitchell, and S. Ebrahim, "Temperature at Birth, Coronary Heart Disease, and Insulin Resistance: Cross Sectional Analyses of the British Women's Heart and Health Study," *Heart* 90 (BMJ Publishing Group, 2004): 381–388.

28. See "Hormones, proteins and carbohydrates in the adaptation to starvation." UCLA Center for Human Nutrition: Basic Principals of Nutrient Metabolism.

29. See G. Holder, J. Moore, J. Tomlinson, L. Shakespeare, P. Clark, and P. Stewart, "Weight Loss Increases 11ß-Hydroxysteroid Dehydrogenase Type 1 Expression in Human Adipose Tissue," *The Journal of Clinical Endocrinology & Metabolism* 89, no. 6 (The Endocrine Society, 2004): 2711–2716.

30. See K. D. Buchanan, R.W. Henry, and R. W. Stout, "Triglyceride Metabolism in Acute Starvation: The Role of Secretin and Glucagon," *European Journal of Clinical Investigation* 6, no. 2 (Blackwell Publishing, March 1976): 179–185.

31. See A. Kubena, F. Duska, I. A. Macdonald, and M. Andel, "Effects of Acute Starvation on Insulin Resistance in Obese Patients With and Without Type 2 Diabetes Mellitus," *Clinical Nutrition* 24, no. 6 (Elsevier, December 2005): 1056–1064.

32. See M. F. Dallman, "Stress Update: Adaptation of the Hypothalamic-Pituitary-Adrenal Axis to Chronic Stress," *Trends in Endocrinology and Metabolism* 4, no. 2 (Elsevier, March 1993): 62–69.

33. See J. Flier, "What's in a Name? In Search of Leptin's Physiologic Role," *The Journal of Clinical Endocrinology & Metabolism* 83, no. 5: (The Endocrine Society, 1998): 1407–1413.

34. See D. Richard and S. Rivest, "Involvement of Corticotropin-Releasing Factor in the Anorexia Induced by Exercise," *Brain Research Bulletin* 25 (Elsevier, July 1990): 169–172.

35. See note 8 above.

36. See M. Schwartz and R. Seeley, "Neuroendocrine Responses to Starvation and Weight Loss," Seminars in Medicine of the Beth Israel Deaconess Medical Center, *The New England Journal of Medicine* 336, no. 25 (June 19, 1997): 1802–1811.

37. See L. S. Brady, M. A. Smith, P. W. Gold, and M. Herkenham, "Altered Expression of Hypothalamic Neuropeptide mRNAs in Food-Restricted and Food-Deprived Rats," *Neuroendocrinology* 52 (1990): 441–447.

38. See H. Inoue, J. Kageyama, K. Hashimoto, S. Suemaru, T. Hattori, and Z. Ota, "Starvation-Induced Changes in Rat Brain Corticotropin-Releasing Factor (CRF) and Pituitary-Adrenocortical Response," *Life Science* 39 (1986): 1161–1166.

39. See D. Deshaies, D. Richard, E. Timofeeva, and F. Picard, "Corticotropin-Releasing Hormone-Binding Protein in Brain and Pituitary of Food-Deprived Bbese (fa/fa) Zucker Rats," *American Journal of Physiology—Regulatory, Integrative, and Comparative Physiology* 277 (American Physiological Society, 1999): R1749–R1759.